Study Guide for

MASTERS, JOHNSON, AND KOLODNY'S

HUMAN SEXUALITY

Study Guide for

MASTERS, JOHNSON, AND KOLODNY'S

HUMAN SEXUALITY

Prepared by
MARVIN R. LEVY
Temple University

LITTLE, BROWN AND COMPANY
BOSTON TORONTO

ISBN 0-316-54992-4

9 8 7 6 5 4 3 2

VB

Published simultaneously in Canada
by Little, Brown & Company (Canada) Limited

Printed in the United States of America

To the Student

This Study Guide is both a workbook to accompany the Masters, Johnson, and Kolodny textbook, Human Sexuality, and a tool to help you integrate the textbook material into a framework you can use to make decisions involving sexuality with increased confidence and consistency.

A functional understanding of human sexuality requires more than the acquisition of factual information. Learning the concepts of sexual behavior and function can open the door to understanding the multidimensional aspects of human sexuality. In addition, a careful and thorough examination of the personal feelings and beliefs that influence the decision-making process is necessary. Therefore, this Study Guide is intended to be more than a means to prepare you for your homework assignments, class presentations, tests, or examinations. It is designed to help you think of human sexuality in a multidimensional way (personal, family, social, biological, psychosocial, behavioral, clinical, cultural, etc.) and to assist you in examining your beliefs about human sexuality in order to clarify your own sexual value system.

The Study Guide begins and ends with a self-administered and scored Sexual Knowledge and Attitude Test. This will enable you to examine the changes in your knowledge during the course by comparing the two sets of scores. You may be surprised to see that not only will your knowledge increase, but some of your attitudes and beliefs about human sexuality will change as well.

You will find that the Study Guide is organized into twenty chapters corresponding to those in the textbook. Each chapter is divided into six parts:

Part I--Learning Objectives
Part II--Important Terms and Names to Know
Part III--Self-Testing: A Programmed Approach
Part IV--Review Quiz
Part V--Clarifying Your Values
Part VI--Answer Key to Review Quiz

You should read the learning objectives for each chapter (Part I) before you read the textbook chapter, then again after you have completed reading the chapter. This will help orient you to the purposes of the material and help you determine your level of achievement following the reading. Gaps will become apparent and you can reread the problematical sections.

Part II highlights the significant terms and names of people covered in the chapter in a sentence completion format. By identifying these particulars, you can develop a more useful foundation for interpersonal communication. Textbook page numbers appear in parentheses following each completion question. The answers appear on the right-hand margin so they can be easily covered up with a strip of heavy paper while you are working on this section. Write the term you think is correct in the blank. Then, immediately check your response by moving the strip of paper down only far enough to expose the correct response. If your response is incorrect, you can review it in the textbook before moving to the next term.

A programmed self-learning format is used in Part III. This will enable you to proceed rapidly over material that is familiar or more easily mastered and concentrate longer on the unfamiliar or more difficult material.

Part IV is a Review Quiz that contains true/false and multiple choice questions (although a few chapters also contain some matching type questions). The correct answers appear in Part VI. The Review Quiz is designed to help you review the material covered in the chapter and serves as a preparation for tests or examinations in class.

The Values Clarification Exercise (Part V) focuses on your value system. It should help you to clarify your attitudes and beliefs about human sexuality, although it won't always help you come up with a "perfect" answer to difficult questions.

Part VI contains the Answer Key to the Review Quiz. It also lists the textbook page numbers for each correct answer. If you missed a question or were not especially confident about your answer, be sure to review the material in the textbook.

One final word--you will find that use of this Study Guide will enhance your understanding of the material presented in each chapter of the text. You may also find that you are better prepared for class discussions and tests. Last, you may find this Study Guide a help in reexamining your sexual values and in being more tolerant of those whose sexual lifestyles differ from your own.

Contents

Study Guide for

MASTERS, JOHNSON, AND KOLODNY'S

HUMAN SEXUALITY

SKAT
SEXUAL KNOWLEDGE AND ATTITUDE TEST
PRETEST

This test is divided into two sections: Part One contains 40 questions on sexual knowledge, and Part Two contains 20 statements about your sexual attitudes.

Instructions for responding to each section are found at the beginning of each section.

Correct answers for the knowledge section (Part One) and scoring directions for the attitude section (Part Two) are found at the end of the Posttest.

It should take you about 30 minutes to complete the SKAT Pretest.

The SKAT Posttest is found at the end of the <u>Study Guide</u>. Instructions for comparing the scores and changes which have occurred are included at the end of the Posttest.

Do not complete the Posttest until you have finished the material in the <u>Study Guide</u> (Chapters 1 - 20).

This test is based on material covered in the textbook and in classroom learning activities. Therefore, as you attend class sessions, read the textbook, and complete the exercises in this <u>Study Guide</u>, your knowledge and attitude about human sexuality will undoubtedly change. By comparing your scores on the Pretest with those on the Posttest, you will be able to measure the extent of these changes.

PART ONE - KNOWLEDGE

<u>True or False</u> (Circle your answer)

T F 1. The more information a person has about human sexuality, the more tolerant he or she is likely to be of the sexual behaviors of others.

T F 2. The external female sex organs include the vagina.

T F 3. The two basic physiologic reactions during human sexual response are myotonia and vasodilation.

T F 4. The third stage of labor involves the delivery of the baby.

T F 5. Health risks during pregnancy are highest in women who are under 18 or over 35 years of age.

T F 6. The genetic codes for male and female sexual differentiation are set in place at the time of conception.

T F 7. The negative messages that children get from their parents when they touch their genitals is considered by many authorities to be unrelated to sexual problems in later years.

T F 8. During early infancy, male babies receive more verbal contact with their mothers than female babies.

T F 9. In romantic love, we tend to immerse ourselves almost completely in another person.

T F 10. Men and women differ significantly in their sexual fantasy patterns.

T F 11. Medical opinion still considers masturbation as a contributing factor in physical and emotional illness.

T F 12. Sex surveys indicate that among young women premarital intercourse is more widespread today than it was 30 years ago.

T F 13. Most biosocial scientists subscribe to the opinion that homosexuality is caused by hormonal mechanisms.

T F 14. Most transvestites have a homosexual orientation.

T F 15. Impotence is probably the most common sexual dysfunction among men in the general population.

T F 16. Erectile dysfunction in men frequently follows a prostatectomy.

T F 17. Most rapes are considered acts of violence.

T F 18. Cultures that are strongly antisexual usually impose stringent censorship practices.

T F 19. Most American clergy are in favor of developing a dialogue about sex.

T F 20. Socially approved sexual contact between children and adults is rare in human history.

Multiple Choice (Circle your answer)

21. The first investigators to utilize direct observations to obtain information about sexual physiology were
    a. Cohen, Rosen, and Goldstein
    b. Masters and Johnson
    c. Kinsey, Pomeroy, and Gebhard
    d. Wilson and Lawson

22. Sperm production begins with the formation of
    a. primary spermatocytes
    b. spermatogonia
    c. spermatids
    d. spermatozoa

23. Ejaculation without orgasm
    a. cannot occur
    b. is common in boys before puberty
    c. can be caused by a diseased prostate
    d. both b and c

24. Induced labor is initiated by giving the pregnant woman
    a. HCG
    b. HMG
    c. DES
    d. oxytocin

25. The exact way that an IUD works is
    a. unknown
    b. interference with ovulation
    c. reduction of cilia movement in the Fallopian tubes
    d. interference with implantation

26. The hormonal differences between girls and boys during childhood are caused by the activity of the
    a. hypothalamus
    b. pituitary
    c. adrenals
    d. gonads

27. The different treatment of boys and girls from the moment of birth is believed to influence
    a. gender identity
    b. gender role
    c. differential socialization
    d. both a and b

28. Gender role socialization is affected by
    a. toys for children
    b. picture books for children
    c. television
    d. all of the above

29. The central feature of love that is lacking in sexual desire is
    a. passion
    b. control
    c. respect
    d. self-fulfillment

30. Sexual fantasies are considered by many sexologists to
   a. be a poor substitute for real experience
   b. permit safe rehearsals of untried behavior
   c. create sexual dysfunction if not acted upon
   d. block the release of inner tensions

31. Research evidence supports the conclusion that
   a. men respond more to erotica than do women
   b. women respond more to erotica than do men
   c. both sexes respond to erotica in similar ways
   d. women respond psychologically and men respond physiologically to all forms of erotica

32. One of the most important considerations for successful sexual contacts is
   a. communication
   b. nongenital pleasuring
   c. genital stimulation
   d. no inhibition about experimenting with new techniques

33. Changes in the law which seem less hostile to the homosexual include
   a. making homosexual acts legal
   b. sentencing the convicted person to a reduced sentence
   c. a ban on employment and housing discrimination
   d. allowing gay men to remain in the military services

34. A paraphilia which focuses on sexual objects rather than sexual acts is
   a. fetishism
   b. exhibitionism
   c. sadomasochism
   d. voyeurism

35. Rigid religious upbringing seems to be a common factor in
   a. secondary impotence
   b. dyspareunia
   c. primary anorgasmia
   d. random anorgasmia

36. The primary cause of sexual problems in both diabetic men and women is
   a. circulatory problems
   b. a form of nerve damage
   c. the effect of insulin injections
   d. of psychogenic origin

37. The key element in coercive sex is
   a. sexual compliance
   b. abuse of physical or social power
   c. sexual harassment
   d. sexual victimization

38. According to United States law
    a. pornography and obscenity are illegal
    b. pornography is legal; obscenity is illegal
    c. pornography is illegal; obscenity is legal
    d. pornography and obscenity are both legal

39. The sexuality position of the majority of Christian religions is based on
    a. scientific evidence
    b. church hierarchy
    c. the Old and New Testaments
    d. all of the above

40. The novelty of new sexual partners is perceived as more sexually stimulating by
    a. industrial societies
    b. preindustrial societies
    c. a few primitive cultures
    d. most cultures

PART TWO - ATTITUDE

Respond to each statement in the following ways:

SA - Circle if you Strongly Agree with the statement.
A - Circle if you Moderately Agree with the statement.
N - Circle if you have no opinion.
D - Circle if you Moderately Disagree with the statement.
SD - Circle if you Strongly Disagree with the statement.

STATEMENTS	LEVEL OF AGREEMENT				
1. Intimacy and emotional involvement should accompany sexual activity.	SA	A	N	D	SD
2. Sexual education should be taught in the public schools.	SA	A	N	D	SD
3. Young people in their reproductive years should have access to contraceptive information and birth control methods.	SA	A	N	D	SD
4. Therapeutic abortions should be available to any woman who desires to terminate a pregnancy.	SA	A	N	D	SD
5. Midwifery and other alternative birthing methods should be available to prospective parents.	SA	A	N	D	SD
6. Childhood sexual experimentation should be viewed as a normal and valuable psychosocial developmental experience.	SA	A	N	D	SD

7.	Premarital coitus is acceptable when two people love each other.	SA	A	N	D	SD
8.	Sexual fantasy should be regarded as a normal and sexually enhancing activity.	SA	A	N	D	SD
9.	Masturbation is an acceptable and healthy form of solitary sexual behavior.	SA	A	N	D	SD
10.	Oral-genital sexual stimulation is neither deviant nor repugnant.	SA	A	N	D	SD
11.	Sexual partners should be willing to try new sexual behaviors.	SA	A	N	D	SD
12.	Extramarital sexual intercourse is permissible under certain situations.	SA	A	N	D	SD
13.	Sexual orientation (preference) should not be a condition for employment, housing, or service (military, ministry).	SA	A	N	D	SD
14.	Prostitution should be decriminalized.	SA	A	N	D	SD
15.	There should be a law to protect women from marital rape.	SA	A	N	D	SD
16.	The penalties for rape should be more equitably applied.	SA	A	N	D	SD
17.	Sexual harassment at work should be against the law.	SA	A	N	D	SD
18.	Pornography should be more clearly defined.	SA	A	N	D	SD
19.	Religion should not get involved with the morality of sexual behavior between adults.	SA	A	N	D	SD
20.	Any activity engaged in by consenting adults, that harms no one, and that is done out of the sight of unwilling viewers, should not be regulated by law.	SA	A	N	D	SD

1

Perspectives on Sexuality

INTRODUCTION

The purpose of this initial chapter is to set the stage for your understanding of human sexuality by focusing upon its multidimensional nature. This is achieved through an examination of the biological, psychosocial, behavioral, clinical, and cultural dimensions of sexuality, as well as historical and research perspectives.

PART I LEARNING OBJECTIVES

At the conclusion of this chapter, you should be able to:

1. Explain the major reasons for studying human sexuality.
2. Describe the role that biological factors play in influencing your sexual desires, functioning, and satisfaction.
3. Identify the primary psychosocial factors that influence your sexuality.
4. Distinguish between the effects of biological and psychosocial forces on sexual behavior.
5. List several obstacles that can lessen the pleasure or spontaneity of sexual encounters.
6. Contrast the changing sexual mores and practices of varying cultures throughout recorded history.
7. Identify the major contributors to contemporary views on human sexuality.
8. Describe the recent trends in sex research.
9. Outline the major components of a research design.
10. List the types of sex research methods, describe each, and give an example of each method.

PART II IMPORTANT TERMS AND NAMES TO KNOW

A. Fill in the missing word or words.

1. __________ refers to a dimension of personality which includes all aspects of being sexual. (2)	sexuality
2. The inner sense a person has of being male or female is called __________ __________. (5)	gender identity
3. Behavior that conveys to others that an individual is either male or female is labelled __________ __________. (7)	gender role
4. A form of sexual behavior which is engaged in for the purpose of having children is called __________ sex. (4)	procreational
5. Sexual activity in the context of emotional involvement and intimacy is known as __________ sex. (4)	relational
6. When we engage in sexual behavior principally to have fun and enjoyment it is referred to as __________ sex. (4)	recreational
7. __________ is sexual activity between a person and a close relative. (8)	incest
8. Sexual intercourse involving a married person with a partner other than his or her spouse is labelled __________. (8)	adultery or extramarital sex
9. Abstention from sexual intercourse is called __________. (9)	celibacy

B. Match the person with the idea, concept, or research

Persons	Idea, Concept, or Research	Key
___1. St. Augustine (9)	a. celibacy not a sign of virtue	Luther
___2. Martin Luther (11)	b. prudery and modesty	Victoria
___3. Queen Victoria (11)	c. psychosexual development	Freud
___4. von Krafft-Ebing (12)	d. sexual response	Masters and Johnson
___5. Sigmund Freud (12)	e. condemnation of sex	Augustine
___6. Havelock Ellis (13)	f. sexual psychopathology	Krafft-Ebing
___7. van de Velde (13)	g. sexual behavior	Kinsey
___8. Alfred Kinsey (14)	h. ideal marriage	van de Velde
___9. Masters and Johnson (14)	i. psychology of sex	Ellis

PART III SELF-TESTING--A PROGRAMMED APPROACH

1. One of the most common misconceptions people have about becoming "better informed" about human sexuality is that it will help to
   a. develop insight into oneself (Go to #2)
   b. encourage more tolerant attitudes toward others (Go to #3)
   c. foster responsible decisions about sexual behavior (Go to #4)
   d. improve skill as a lover (Go to #5)

2. Sex education can help people understand themselves and thereby gain self-insight and self-knowledge. It is not a misconception. You are incorrect. (Go to #5)

3. Learning about sexuality in an objective fashion often helps people become more aware and more tolerant of the behaviors of others. It is not a misconception; you are incorrect. (Go to #5)

4. Reasoned decisions and responsible interpersonal sexual behavior are outgrowths of sexual knowledge. It is not a misconception; you are incorrect. (Go to #5)

5. A common misconception that many people hold is that if a person becomes better informed about sexuality, he or she will find greater pleasure in sex and become more adept at giving pleasure to others (i.e., by being a better lover). Although this can certainly happen, it is not due to knowledge alone but to a combination of forces. You are correct in identifying this idea as a misconception. (Go to #6)

6. Gender identity is shaped primarily by
   a. biological forces (Go to #7)
   b. psychosocial forces (Go to #8)
   c. behavioral forces (Go to #9)
   d. cultural forces (Go to #10)

7. Biological forces largely control reproduction and sexual functioning but not gender identity. You are incorrect. (Go to #8)

8. Psychosocial forces such as the ways in which our parents, peers, and teachers react to us help shape our view of ourselves as males or females. You are correct. (Go to #11)

9. Sexual behavior is a product of both biological and psychosocial forces. Our gender identity can be quite different from the way in which we act. You are incorrect. (Go to #8)

10. Cultural attitudes tend to foster gender role stereotypes rather than our personal sense of maleness or femaleness. You are incorrect. (Go to #8)

11. The rebirth of humanism and the arts during the Renaissance contributed to
    a. a more rigid set of sexual restrictions (Go to #12)
    b. adherence to the practice of courtly love (Go to #13)
    c. a loosening of sexual restrictions (Go to #14)
    d. the view that chastity and celibacy were virtues (Go to #15)

12. Rigid sexual restrictions were manifest during the early Christian era. You are incorrect. (Go to #14)

13. Courtly love emerged as a new code of acceptable behavior during the Medieval period. You are incorrect. (Go to #14)

14. The Renaissance in Europe during the sixteenth and seventeenth centuries encouraged a relaxation of the sexual restrictions promulgated by the Church and reduced the necessity to adhere to the standards of courtly love. You are correct. (Go to #16)

15. Chastity and celibacy were viewed as virtues prior to the Reformation. You are incorrect. (Go to #14)

16. The most controversial type of sex research continues to be
    a. observational studies (Go to #17)
    b. interview surveys (Go to #18)
    c. case studies (Go to #19)
    d. questionnaire surveys (Go to #20)

17. Due to the personal nature of human sexuality, observational studies are often subject to public and political pressures. You are correct. (Go to Part IV)

18. Interview surveys have limitations but are less controversial than direct observation by a human observer or instrument to record the event(s). You are incorrect. (Go to #17)

19. Case studies focus on a limited number of subjects who manifest a similar behavior (e.g., rapists, nymphomaniacs). While the behavior being investigated may be controversial, the technique is commonly accepted. You are incorrect. (Go to #17)

20. Survey research is the least controversial method employed in sex research, especially when it is conducted by questionnaire. You are incorrect. (Go to #17)

PART IV REVIEW QUIZ

A. <u>True or False</u>

___ 1. Biological factors are those which not only shape our gender identity but also influence our gender role.

___ 2. Misinformation about sex can sometimes lead to sexual problems.

___ 3. Our early sexual attitudes formed in childhood and adolescence are usually outgrown in our adult lives.

___ 4. Psychosocial factors largely control our sexual attitudes and beliefs.

___ 5. Sexual behavior is the product of gender identity and endocrine function.

___ 6. Sex was strongly condemned in the early theological writings of St. Augustine.

___ 7. Applying research findings from a sample to a larger group is called sample selection.

___ 8. The accuracy of a measurement procedure depends on its validity, and its consistency depends on its reliability.

___ 9. When one factor in a research study is manipulated by the investigator under carefully controlled conditions, the method is known as experimental research.

___ 10. Ethics dictates that when conducting sex research, the purposes and procedures of the research should be explained to prospective participants.

B. <u>Multiple Choice--Select the Best Answer.</u>

___ 11. Our sexual heritage can be understood by studying sexuality from which of the following perspectives?
   a. biological and behavioral
   b. psychosocial and cultural
   c. clinical and historical
   d. all of the above

___ 12. Learning about sexuality enables you to
a. become a better lover
b. find more sexual pleasure
c. have deeper insight into self and others
d. all of the above

___ 13. Sex shared with a cared-for person is called
a. relational sex
b. procreational sex
c. recreational sex
d. reciprocal sex

___ 14. Certain obstacles can lessen spontaneity of our sexual encounters, such as
a. illness
b. drugs
c. anxiety
d. all of the above

___ 15. The public expression of gender identity is known as
a. gender role
b. gender orientation
c. gender preference
d. none of the above

___ 16. Sex was recognized as a creative and pleasurable force in
a. Plato's Republic
b. Song of Solomon
c. Letters of Paul
d. Confessions of St. Augustine

___ 17. Advocates of the Protestant Reformation (e.g., Luther, Calvin) sanctioned
a. more restrictions on sexual behaviors than the Catholic Church
b. the same number of restrictions on sexual behaviors as the Catholic Church
c. less negative sexual attitudes than the Catholic Church
d. similar views on chastity as the Catholic Church

___ 18. Extremes in prudery and modesty prevailed during the
a. Victorian era
b. Renaissance
c. Medieval period
d. Reformation

___ 19. A detailed classification of sexual disorders first appeared during the
a. 17th Century
b. 18th Century
c. 19th Century
d. 20th Century

___ 20. The centrality of sexuality to human existence was portrayed most effectively by
a. St. Augustine
b. von Krafft-Ebing
c. Havelock Ellis
d. Sigmund Freud

___ 21. The first investigators to utilize direct observations to obtain information about sexual physiology were
a. Cohen, Rosen, and Goldstein
b. Masters and Johnson
c. Kinsey, Pomeroy, and Gebhard
d. Wilson and Lawson

___ 22. Which of the following areas of sex research has been largely neglected by investigators?
a. homosexuality
b. disability
c. contraceptive practices
d. childhood sexuality

___ 23. The decisions made in the course of planning a research study are collectively referred to as the
a. research design
b. source of information
c. sampling strategy
d. data analyses

___ 24. Research which studies the distribution of a particular behavior in a population is
a. survey research
b. observational research
c. clinical research
d. experimental research

___ 25. A systematic source of error in research is called
a. inconsistency
b. homogeneity
c. bias
d. placebo effect

PART V CLARIFYING YOUR VALUES

Every person has unique sexual feelings, attitudes, and beliefs because they are processed through an intensely personal perspective. This perspective comes from a host of sources, some internal and others external to the individual. The activity which follows below is designed to give you an opportunity to examine some of these sources.

Considering your own personal beliefs about human sexuality, indicate the degree to which each of the dimensions shown in the grid has influenced your beliefs by placing a check-mark under the appropriate column. The following scale is used to express the degree of influence:

VS = Very Significant Influence
SS = Somewhat Significant Influence
NS = Not a Significant Influence

PERSPECTIVES ON SEXUALITY

Sources	Dimensions														
	Biological			Psychosocial			Behavioral			Clinical			Cultural		
	VS	SS	NS	VS	SS	NS	VS	SS	NS	VS	SS	NS	VS	SS	NS
Personal Experience															
Family Patterns															
Peer Standards															
Historical Events															
Religious Views															
Research Findings															

PART VI ANSWER KEY TO REVIEW QUIZ

1. False. See text p. 5.
2. True. See text p. 2.
3. False. See text p. 5.
4. True. See text p. 5.
5. False. See text p. 5.
6. True. See text p. 9.
7. False. See text p. 18.
8. True. See text p. 20.
9. True. See text p. 21.
10. True. See text p. 20.
11. (d) See text p. 1.
12. (c) See text p. 2.
13. (a) See text p. 4.
14. (d) See text p. 5.
15. (a) See text p. 7.
16. (b) See text p. 8.
17. (c) See text p. 11.
18. (a) See text p. 11.
19. (c) See text p. 12.
20. (d) See text p. 12.
21. (b) See text pp. 15-16.
22. (d) See text p. 17.
23. (a) See text pp. 17-20.
24. (a) See text p. 20.
25. (c) See text pp. 21-22.

2

Sexual Anatomy

INTRODUCTION

This chapter presents a concise discussion of male and female sexual anatomy. It includes both reproductive organs and structures that have erotic significance.

PART I LEARNING OBJECTIVES

At the conclusion of this chapter, you should be able to:

1. Explain why people have mixed feelings about their sexual body parts.
2. Identify a source of negative attitudes about sexual anatomy for both sexes.
3. Label parts of the male sexual anatomy, including the external and internal sex organs.
4. Label parts of the female sexual anatomy, including the external and internal sex organs.
5. Describe the process of egg and sperm formation.
6. List and discuss the structures of potential sexual pleasure (i.e., erogenous areas) in both sexes.

PART II IMPORTANT TERMS AND NAMES TO KNOW

Fill in the missing word or words.

1. The __________ are the external sex organs in the female. (31) — vulva

2. The area over the pubic bone of the female is the __________ __________. (31) — mons veneris

3. __________ __________ are the outer folds of skin on either side of the urethral and vaginal openings. The inner lips are called the __________ __________. (31)

   labia majora
   labia minora

4. The __________ of the female is the erectile body comprised of three parts: the __________, __________, and __________. (32-33)

   clitoris
   hood, glans, shaft

5. Internal branches of the clitoral shaft in females and corpora cavernosa in males which attach to the bony pelvis are the __________. (33)

   crura

6. Accumulation of secretions, dead cells, and bacteria under the foreskin of the penis and the hood of the clitoris is called __________. (34)

   smegma

7. The __________ is the area of skin between the vagina and the anus. (34)

   perineum

8. A thin tissue covering the opening of the vagina is the __________. (35)

   hymen

9. The __________ is a muscle which encircles and supports the vagina; the muscle that supports the entrance to the vagina is the __________. (36)

   pubococcygeus
   bulbocavernosus

10. The hollow pear-shaped muscular internal female genital organ is the __________. (38)

    uterus

11. The __________ is the inner lining of the uterus; the muscular part is the __________. (38)

    endometrium
    myometrium

12. __________ __________ are transport ducts for eggs. (39)

    Fallopian tubes

13. __________ is the process by which each immature egg divides. (39)

    meiosis

14. An __________ is a mature egg cell; two or more are __________. (39) — ovum, ova

15. The __________ __________ is the part of the ovarian follicle left in the ovary after an egg is expelled. (39) — corpus luteum

16. __________ __________ is a jelly-like material surrounding the mature egg. (39) — zona pellucida

17. A circular area of dark skin around the nipple is called the __________. (42) — areola

18. __________ is an unusual enlargement of the breast. (43) — macromastia

19. The cylinder of erectile tissue along the underside of the penis which contains the urethra is the __________ __________. (44) — corpus spongiosum

20. The __________ __________ is comprised of two cylindrical bodies of erectile tissue in the penis and the clitoris. (44) — corpora cavernosa

21. The head of the penis or clitoris is called the __________. (44) — glans

22. The __________ __________ is the rim of tissue that separates the glans from the shaft of the penis. The __________ is the small triangular fold of skin on the underside of the penis. (44) — coronal ridge, frenulum

23. __________ is a freely movable piece of skin tissue which covers the penis and clitoris. (44) — foreskin

24. The __________ is a thin loose sac of skin that contains the testes. (48) — scrotum

25.	__________, often called the male hormone, is actually secreted by both sexes. (48)	testosterone
26.	__________ __________ produce hormones in the testes. (48)	Leydig cells
27.	Microscopic tube-shaped structures in the testes that produce sperm are called __________ __________. (48)	seminiferous tubules
28.	When mature spermatogonia undergo meitotic division __________ __________ and __________ __________ are formed. The latter will divide into __________. (48)	primary spermatocytes secondary spermatocytes spermatids
29.	The chemical reservoir in the head of spermatozoa is called the __________. (40)	acrosome
30.	Sperm cells mature in the __________, which is a tubing network folded against the back surface of each testis. (50)	epididymis
31.	The __________ __________ are two tube-like structures that transport sperm from the testes. (50)	vas deferens
32.	The __________ __________ is located directly below the bladder and surrounds the urethra. It secretes part of the seminal fluid. (50-51)	prostate gland
33.	__________ __________ is the thick white, yellow, or gray liquid portion of the male ejaculate. (51)	seminal fluid
34.	A pair of pouch-like bodies, the __________ __________, empty into the __________ __________ and provide the major portion of fluid in the ejaculate. (51)	seminal vesicles ejaculatory ducts
35.	The __________ __________ are two pea-sized structures that produce the pre-ejaculatory fluid. (51)	Cowpers glands

36. __________ is a condition of male breast enlargement. gynecomastia

(51)

PART III SELF-TESTING--A PROGRAMMED APPROACH

1. The external sex organs of the female called vulva consist of
   a. mons, labia, and vagina (Go to #2)
   b. mons, labia, vagina, and perineum (Go to #3)
   c. mons, labia, clitoris, vagina, and perineum (Go to #4)
   d. mons, labia, clitoris, and perineum (Go to #5)

2. The vagina is principally an internal organ. The clitoris and perineum, which are external organs, were omitted. You are incorrect. (Go to #5)

3. This response omits the clitoris, which is an external sex organ; it includes the vagina, an internal organ. You are incorrect. (Go to #5)

4. The inclusion of the vagina, which is an internal organ, made this choice incorrect. All the other structures are external organs. (Go to #5)

5. You are correct since all the other choices were incorrect due primarily to the fact that the vagina, which is an internal organ, was included in the other choices. (Go to #6)

6. Kegel exercises are
   a. done by consciously contracting the pelvic muscles that support the uterus (Go to #7)
   b. designed to prevent objects from being inserted into the vagina (Go to #8)
   c. useful in improving a woman's sense of self-awareness (Go to #9)
   d. capable of improving a woman's sexual responsivity (Go to #10)

7. The muscles which are contracted are the pubococcygeus and bulbocavernosus muscles which support the vagina, not the uterus. You are incorrect. (Go to #9)

8. Contractions of the vaginal muscles, especially the bulbocavernosus, can tighten the entrance to the vagina; however, Kegel exercises are not used to create uncontrolled spasms which impede penetration of the vagina. You are incorrect. (Go to #9)

9. Kegel exercises strengthen the muscular contractions of the pelvic muscles but are also found to improve and heighten a woman's sense of self-awareness. You are correct. (Go to #11)

10. There is no clearcut evidence at this point in time to support the belief that the practice of Kegel's exercises will improve sexual responsivity. You are incorrect. (Go to #9)

11. Sperm production begins with the formation of
    a. primary spermatocytes (Go to #12)
    b. spermatogonia (Go to #13)
    c. spermatids (Go to #14)
    d. spermatozoa (Go to #15)

12. Primary spermatocytes and secondary spermatocytes are transformed from spermatogonia by a process known as meiotic division. You are incorrect. (Go to #13)

13. Spermatogonia are the primitive cells which are produced in the seminiferous tubules. They are the initial form of spermatogenesis. You are correct. (Go to #16)

14. Spermatids are actually the fourth generation in sperm production. They are transformed from secondary spermatocytes. You are incorrect. (Go to #13)

15. Spermatozoa are the mature sperm cells which are the last in a series of transformations beginning with primitive spermatogonia in the seminiferous tubules. You are incorrect. (Go to #13)

16. Erectile tissue is found in all of the following structures except
    a. corpus spongiosum (Go to #17)
    b. corpora cavernosa (Go to #18)
    c. corpus uterus (Go to #19)
    d. clitoris (Go to #20)

17. The corpus spongiosum is similar in structure to the corpora cavernosa; both consist of erectile tissue with irregular sponge-like networks of connective tissue interspersed with many small thin-walled blood vessels. You are incorrect. (Go to #19)

18. The corpora cavernosa are two cylinders in the penis which are similar in structure to the corpus spongiosum. They all contain erectile tissue. You are incorrect. (Go to #19)

19. The uterus consists of several parts, one of which comprises the main portion and is called the corpus or body. The muscular component is the myometrium. The corpus contains no erectile tissue. You are correct; it is the exception.

20. The clitoris is derived embryologically from the same tissues as the penis and does become engorged when stimulated. It is not, however, a miniature penis. You are incorrect. (Go to #19)

PART IV REVIEW QUIZ

A. True or False

___ 1. Many people have inaccurate information or negative feelings about their sexual anatomy.

___ 2. The words we use to talk about sexual anatomy often convey a negative attitude.

___ 3. Most of us were taught in early childhood that the sex organs were unclean.

___ 4. The mons veneris is one of the external female structures that is relatively devoid of nerve endings.

___ 5. An intact hymen is proof of virginity.

___ 6. The finger-like projections at the end of the oviducts are called cilia.

___ 7. The advantages of circumcision are primarily related to cleanliness and disease prevention.

___ 8. Concern over penis size is common in males of all ages.

___ 9. The prostate gland, the largest of the male sex organs, produces the major portion of the fluid ejaculate.

___ 10. Many men and women have no idea of the location of the female clitoris.

B. Multiple Choice--Select the Best Answer

___ 11. The area over the pubic bone which consists of a cushion of fatty tissue covered by skin and pubic hair in women is the
- a. labia
- b. mons
- c. hood
- d. groin

___ 12. Labia minora form into a fold of skin just above the clitoris called the
- a. clitoral hood
- b. clitoral glans
- c. clitoral shaft
- d. crura

___ 13. Bartholin's glands
- a. neutralize the pH of the vagina
- b. contribute significantly to vaginal lubrication
- c. stimulate the clitoris
- d. have no clearly understood function

___ 14. The clitoris is located
- a. at the opening of the vagina
- b. directly next to the hymen
- c. between the vaginal and the urethral openings
- d. beneath the point where the top of the inner lips meet

___ 15. The hairless area of skin between the bottom of the labia and the anus is the
- a. perineum
- b. periteneum
- c. perimetrium
- d. perimastium

___ 16. The hymen is
a. a thin membrane covering the vaginal opening
b. a protection from disease organisms entering the vagina
c. a ligament that supports the labia
d. a covering for the clitoris

___ 17. The bottom part of the uterus is the
a. fundus
b. corpus
c. cervix
d. isthmus

___ 18. The inside lining of the uterus is called the
a. ectometrium
b. myometrium
c. endometrium
d. mesometrium

___ 19. A newborn female has approximately __________ immature eggs.
a. 100,000
b. 200,000
c. 300,000
d. 400,000

___ 20. Eggs are usually fertilized in the
a. uterus
b. ovaries
c. Fallopian tubes
d. graffian follicle

___ 21. The average size of a flaccid penis is just under
a. six inches/15 centimeters
b. five inches/13 centimeters
c. four inches/10 centimeters
d. three inches/8 centimeters

___ 22. Smegma is made up of
a. oily secretions
b. sweat
c. bacteria
d. all of the above

___ 23. The chemical reservoir (acrosome) of the sperm is found in the
a. head
b. midpiece
c. tail
d. all of the above

___ 24. Sperm cells spend several weeks maturing in the
   a. seminiferous tubules
   b. epididymis
   c. vas deferens
   d. seminal vesicles

___ 25. A condition where one or both of a male's breasts become enlarged is called
   a. mastitis
   b. macromastia
   c. gynecomastia
   d. mammary defeminization

C. Match the numbers in the diagram with the list of sexual organs

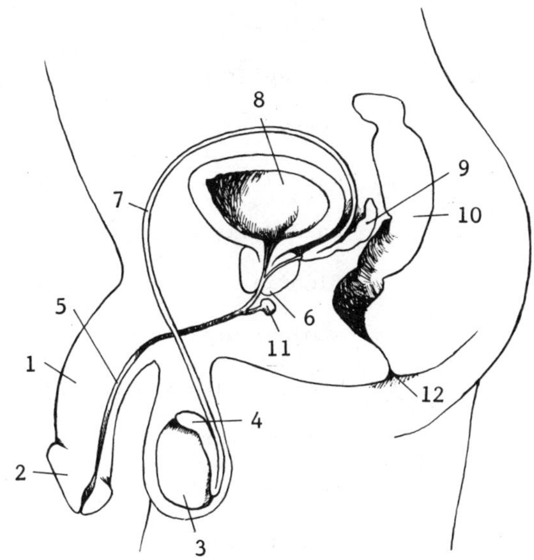

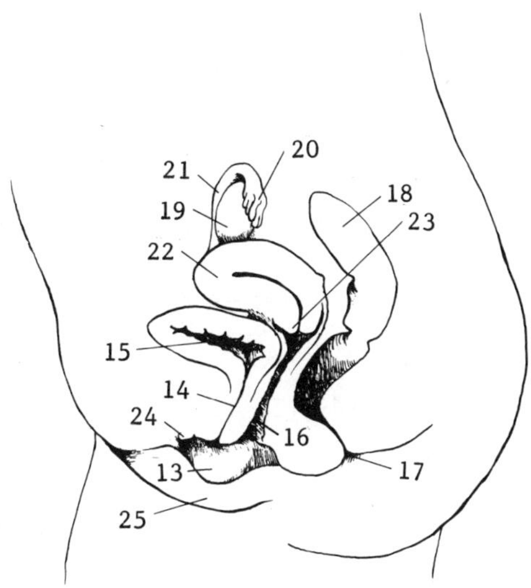

Number on Diagram	List of Sexual Organs
1. ______	a. female anus
2. ______	b. clitoris
3. ______	c. male anus
4. ______	d. Cowpers gland
5. ______	e. male urinary bladder
6. ______	f. female urethra
7. ______	g. glans
8. ______	h. labia majora
9. ______	i. vas deferens
10. ______	j. ovary
11. ______	k. cervix
12. ______	l. epididymis
13. ______	m. fimbria
14. ______	n. seminal vesicle
15. ______	o. female urinary bladder
16. ______	p. male urethra
17. ______	q. penis
18. ______	r. female rectum
19. ______	s. testis
20. ______	t. vagina
21. ______	u. labia minora
22. ______	v. prostate
23. ______	w. Fallopian tube
24. ______	x. male rectum
25. ______	y. uterus

PART V CLARIFYING YOUR VALUES

An erogenous area--like beauty--is in the eye of the beholder! Some of us can get turned on sexually by gentle stroking of the skin on our back; others will find it relaxing but not sensuous; some people may find that it tickles and is not erotic. What each of us values sexually is due to a variety of factors, especially those affecting our feelings and behaviors. Most of us recognize that our values on issues fall somewhere along a continuum or range represented by opposite extremes at each end.

Several continua are presented below. Each represents a part of the sexual anatomy which can be the source of erotic pleasure to some people. Identify the degree to which you consider the anatomical part to be erogenous for you by placing an "X" on the continuum which most accurately reflects your feeling. In the "Comment" section, briefly describe your reasons for holding this position.

<u>Breasts</u> (female)

-10	0	+10
A Turn-off	Neutral	Ecstasy

<u>Breasts</u> (male)

-10	0	+10
A Turn-off	Neutral	Ecstasy

<u>Insides of thighs</u> (female)

-10	0	+10
A Turn-off	Neutral	Ecstasy

<u>Insides of thighs</u> (male)

-10	0	+10
A Turn-off	Neutral	Ecstasy

Buttocks (female)

-10	0	+10
A Turn-off	Neutral	Ecstasy

Buttocks (male)

-10	0	+10
A Turn-off	Neutral	Ecstasy

Mouth (female)

-10	0	+10
A Turn-off	Neutral	Ecstasy

Mouth (male)

-10	0	+10
A Turn-off	Neutral	Ecstasy

Perineum (female)

-10	0	+10
A Turn-off	Neutral	Ecstasy

Perineum (male)

-10	0	+10
A Turn-off	Neutral	Ecstasy

COMMENTS

Breasts (female)

Breasts (male)

Inside of thighs (female)

Inside of thighs (male)

Buttocks (female)

Buttocks (male)

Mouth (female)

Mouth (male)

Perineum (female)

Perineum (male)

PART VI ANSWER KEY TO REVIEW QUIZ

1. True. See text p. 29.
2. True. See text p. 30.
3. True. See text pp. 30-31.
4. False. See text p. 31.
5. False. See text p. 36.
6. False. See text p. 39.
7. True. See text p. 46.
8. True. See text pp. 46-48.
9. False. See text p. 51.
10. True. See text p. 31.
11. (b) See text p. 31.
12. (a) See text p. 33.
13. (d) See text p. 32.
14. (d) See text p. 32.
15. (a) See text p. 34.
16. (a) See text p. 35.
17. (c) See text p. 36.
18. (c) See text p. 38.
19. (d) See text p. 39.
20. (c) See text p. 39.
21. (c) See text p. 48.
22. (d) See text p. 44.
23. (a) See text p. 50.
24. (b) See text p. 50.
25. (c) See text p. 51.

ANSWER KEY TO DIAGRAMS

1. q
2. g
3. s
4. l
5. p
6. v
7. i
8. e
9. n
10. x
11. d
12. c
13. u
14. f
15. o
16. t
17. a
18. r
19. j
20. m
21. w
22. y
23. k
24. b
25. h

3
Sexual Physiology

INTRODUCTION

Chapter Three focuses on the functions of our sexual anatomy. It includes a description of the sources of sexual arousal, the sexual response cycle, common myths about sexual response, hormonal regulation of sexual function and behavior, and menstruation.

PART I LEARNING OBJECTIVES

At the conclusion of this chapter, you should be able to:

1. Identify the sources of sexual arousal.
2. Explain the two basic physiologic reactions during human sexual response.
3. List and contrast the physiologic changes that occur during the four phases of human sexual response.
4. Discuss the controversies that exist about the nature of female orgasms.
5. Describe several commonly held myths about sexual response.
6. List the sex hormones and discuss their effects on sexual function.
7. Identify and explain the three phases of the menstrual cycle.
8. Describe the two most common problems related to menstruation experienced by women.
9. Examine your belief about sexual activity during menstruation and contrast it with those beliefs held by others.
10. Analyze the strengths and weaknesses of the menstrual cycle research conducted in the last decade.

PART II IMPORTANT TERMS AND NAMES TO KNOW

A. Fill in the missing word or words.

1. __________ is an increased amount of blood concentrated in body tissues. (57) — vasocongestion

2. An involuntary contraction of a muscle is called __________. (57) — myotonia

3. The __________ phase of the human sexual response cycle is the first of four phases described by Masters and Johnson. (57-58) — excitement

4. The passing of a fluid through a membrane as in the lubrication of the vagina is known as __________. (59) — transudation

5. The __________ phase of the human sexual response cycle is a time where high levels of sexual arousal are maintained and intensified. (62) — plateau

6. The swelling of tissues due to vasocongestion in the outer third of the vagina is called the __________ __________. (62) — orgasmic platform

7. __________ __________ is a reddish, spotty skin color generally occurring during the late excitement or early plateau phase. (64) — sex flush

8. An __________ is a sudden discharge of accumulated sexual tension and is the shortest phase of the human sexual response cycle. (65) — orgasm

9. The feeling or sensation a man experiences when he has passed the point where ejaculation can be controlled is called __________ __________. (66) — ejaculatory inevitability

10. The last phase of the human sexual response cycle is called the __________ phase. (68) — resolution

11. The potential ability of women to have a series of identifiable orgasms without dropping below the plateau level is known as being __________. (68) — multiorgasmic

12. The __________ __________ immediately following ejaculation is characterized by a male's inability to have a further ejaculation. (70) — refractory period

13. A __________ __________ is an ejaculation during sleep. (71) — nocturnal emission or wet dream

14. __________ are chemical substances produced by endocrine glands. (72) — hormones

15. __________ is the most important hormone in sexual function as it is the principal biologic determinant of the sex drive. (72) — testosterone

16. The hormone which maintains the lining of the vagina, produces breast growth, and is important in controlling the menstrual cycle is __________. (72) — estrogen

17. __________ is a hormone that is produced in high levels by the corpus luteum and is present in high levels during pregnancy. (72) — progesterone

18. The __________ gland functions like a relay station which at the direction of the __________ secretes several hormones important to sexual functioning. (72-73) — pituitary; hypothalamus

19. The hypothalamus produces __________ __________ __________ that controls hormones of the pituitary gland. (73) — gonadotropin releasing hormone

20. __________ hormone stimulates the Leydig cells to manufacture testosterone. (73) — luteinizing

21. The __________ __________ hormone stimulates the production of sperm cells in the testes and prepares the ovaries for ovulation. (73) — follicle stimulating

22. __________ is the flow of blood that occurs about once a month in most women between the ages of 12 and 48. (74) — menstruation

23. The __________ phase of the menstrual cycle is the one in which ovarian follicles begin to mature. (75) — follicular

24. The __________ phase is characterized by the release of an egg from an ovary. (76) — ovulatory

25. The time from immediately after ovulation until the start of menstruation is called the __________ phase. (76) — luteal

26. Painful menstruation is known as __________. (78) — dysmenorrhea

27. A condition known as the __________ __________ may occur 2 or 3 days before menstrual flow and is marked by feelings of tension and irritability. (78) — premenstrual syndrome

B. Match the name(s) with the idea, concept, or research

Names	Idea, Concept, or Research	Key
___1. Masters and Johnson (57)	a. phases of sexual response cycle	Masters and Johnson
___2. Sigmund Freud (67-68)	b. analysis of women's views on own sexual responsivity	Hite
___3. Alfred Kinsey (71)	c. clitoral orgasms were evidence of psychological immaturity	Freud
___4. Katherine Dalton (78)	d. females have orgasms in sleep	Kinsey
___5. Shere Hite (68)	e. premenstrual and menstrual phases behaviors	Dalton

PART III SELF-TESTING--A PROGRAMMED APPROACH

1. The findings of the Masters and Johnson investigation of human physiology indicated the typical human sexual response pattern could be described as a cycle with four phases in the following sequence:
   a. plateau, excitement, arousal, orgasm (Go to #2)
   b. arousal, excitement, plateau, orgasm (Go to #3)
   c. excitement, orgasm, plateau, resolution (Go to #4)
   d. excitement, plateau, orgasm, resolution (Go to #5)

2. Plateau is out of sequence and there is no arousal phase; resolution is missing. You are incorrect. (Go to #5)

3. Arousal, although used synonymously with sexual excitement, is not a separate phase; resolution phase is missing. You are incorrect. (Go to #5)

4. Excitement typically occurs first, however orgasm more typically follows the plateau phase rather than precedes it. You are incorrect. (Go to #5)

5. The pattern is typical. You are correct. (Go to #6)

6. The two basic physiologic reactions during human sexual response are
   a. vasodilation and carpopedal spasm (Go to #7)
   b. myotonia and tachycardia (Go to #8)
   c. vasocongestion and increased neuromuscular tension (Go to #9)
   d. transudation and myotonia (Go to #10)

7. Vasodilatation may be caused by certain drugs or alcoholic beverages. This interferes with the normal physiologic response, which is congestion of blood in the genitals and female breasts. Carpopedal spasm may occur but is only one form of neuromuscular tension. You are incorrect. (Go to #9)

8. Myotonia is one of the basic physiologic reactions; however, although an increase in heart rate (tachycardia) can and often does occur, it is not a basic physiologic reaction. You are incorrect. (Go to #9)

9. Congestion of blood (vasocongestion) and increased neuromuscular tension are the two basic physiologic reactions during human sexual response. You are correct. (Go to #11)

10. Transudation can occur due to vasocongestion but it is too limited a form of physiologic response to be considered a basic reaction. Myotonia is the second mechanism; however, you are incorrect. (Go to #9)

11. The first signs of sexual excitement in men and women are
    a. erection of the penis and vaginal lubrication (Go to #12)
    b. testes increase in size and vagina expands (Go to #13)
    c. nipple erection occurs in both sexes (Go to #14)
    d. testes are elevated and breasts increase in size (Go to #15)

12. The erect penis and the moistened vagina are the physical hallmarks of sexual excitation and usually occur due to vasocongestion very early in sexual stimulation. You are correct. (Go to #16)

13. The testes do increase in size and the inner two-thirds of the vagina expand during the excitement phase but these usually <u>follow</u> the vasocongestion reaction which produces erection of the penis and lubrication of the vagina. You are incorrect. (Go to #12)

14. Nipple erection usually occurs in the female and in some men during the excitement phase. These responses, however, occur later in the excitement phase than erection of the penis and lubrication of the vagina. You are incorrect. (Go to #12)

15. The testes are partially drawn toward the body by a shortening of the spermatic cords and there may be a small increase in female breast size, but these occur late in the exitement phase. You are incorrect. (Go to #12)

16. The major difference between male and female sexual response immediately following orgasm is the fact that
    a. all women experience multiple orgasms (Go to #17)
    b. men have a refractory period; women do not (Go to #18)
    c. women need constant physical stimulation to keep aroused (Go to #19)
    d. women do not experience orgasm during sleep (Go to #20)

17. All women have the physical capacity of being multiorgasmic; however, most women infrequently are. You are incorrect. (Go to #18)

18. The refractory period phenomenon which requires a recovery time before another ejaculation is possible occurs in males, not in females. It is the major difference between the sexes immediately following orgasm. You are correct.

19. Women tend to remain physiologically capable of unlimited orgasmic potential. Their sexual arousal, however, depends on effective sexual stimulation and sexual interest. These usually involve a total response to several stimuli, not just to those of physical origin. You are incorrect. (Go to #18)

20. One of the common misconceptions held about the differences between men and women is that only young men experience orgasm during sleep. Almost 30 years ago, Kinsey reported that females can also experience orgasm during sleep. You are incorrect. (Go to #18)

PART IV REVIEW QUIZ

<u>A. True or False</u>

___ 1. Unexpected sexual arousal is normal and happens to most of us at one time or another.

___ 2. The phases of the human sexual response cycle are clearly distinct from one another.

___ 3. The physiology of sexual response is the same for heterosexuals and homosexuals.

___ 4. Excitation can be a result of sexual stimulation which may be physical or psychological.

___ 5. Vaginal lubrication is produced by the vasocongestion in the walls of the vagina.

___ 6. The amount of lubrication is a good indicator of the woman's level of arousal.

___ 7. The color change in the labia minora during the plateau phase will invariably be followed by orgasm if effective sexual stimulation continues.

___ 8. Since women do not ejaculate, they are incapable of a true orgasm.

___ 9. All females are physiologically capable of being multiorgasmic.

___ 10. Most women are regular enough in their menstrual cycle that they can consistently and accurately predict the length of each cycle on the basis of their past pattern of cycle lengths.

B. <u>Multiple Choice--Select the Best Answer</u>

___ 11. Men have about ______ erections during a night's sleep and women have a similar number of episodes of vaginal lubrication during sleep.
a. 2
b. 6
c. 10
d. 12

___ 12. The first direct laboratory observation of human sexual physiology was conducted during the
a. 1940s
b. 1950s
c. 1960s
d. 1970s

___ 13. The initial physiological sexual response to sexual stimulation is
a. myotonia
b. tachycardia
c. hyperventilation
d. vasocongestion

___ 14. The first signs of sexual excitation in the female start ______________ after the onset of sexual stimulation.
a. 10 to 30 seconds
b. 30 to 60 seconds
c. 1 to 3 minutes
d. 3 to 5 minutes

___ 15. Changes which occur in women during the excitement phase include
a. orgasmic platform
b. clitoral retraction
c. transudation
d. clitoral increase in size

___ 16. The duration of the plateau phase
a. is briefer in men than in women
b. varies widely
c. is always more than 5 minutes
d. is briefer in women than in men

___ 17. The swelling of the tissues in the outer third of the vagina during the plateau phase narrows the opening of the vagina by _____ percent or more.
a. 90
b. 70
c. 50
d. 30

___ 18. The labia minora enlarge dramatically in the plateau phase
a. pushing the outer lips apart
b. making the entry to the introitus more difficult
c. increasing vaginal lubrication
d. exposing more of the clitoral shaft

___ 19. The reddish, spotty skin color change that resembles measles (the sex flush) generally
a. occurs across the upper back and shoulders
b. begins along the medial axis of the neck and spreads laterally
c. begins just below the breast bone and spreads to the chest
d. occurs in the pelvic area and spreads to the thighs and hips

___ 20. Nongenital physiological responses in both men and women include
a. an increased heart rate
b. an increase in blood pressure
c. an increased rate of breathing
d. all of the above

___ 21. Intensity of orgasm can be affected by
a. physical factors
b. psychological factors
c. physical and psychological factors
d. none of the above

___ 22. The belief that women didn't have orgasms reflected a
a. researcher bias
b. sampling bias
c. cultural bias
d. volunteer bias

___ 23. Orgasms in men occur in _____ distinct stage(s)

a. one
b. two
c. three
d. four

___ 24. Ejaculation without orgasm

a. cannot occur
b. is common in boys before puberty
c. can be caused by a diseased prostate
d. both b and c above

___ 25. Which involuntary response may be misinterpreted by a sexual partner as discomfort or displeasure?

a. muscle spasms
b. facial grimacing
c. hyperventilation
d. body rigidity

___ 26. What phenomenon prevents males from being multiorgasmic?

a. lack of adequate sexual stimulation after orgasm
b. lack of sexual interest after orgasm
c. need for physiological recovery period
d. need for a multiorgasmic partner

___ 27. What two problems related to menstruation are most common among women?

a. dysmenorrhea and dramatic mood alteration
b. dysmenorrhea and premenstrual syndrome
c. premenstrual syndrome and amenorrhea
d. amenorrhea and dramatic mood alteration

C. Matching

	Sexual Response Phase		Sexual Physiology
___ 28.	Excitement	a.	muscular contractions
___ 29.	Plateau	b.	vaginal lubrication and penile erection
___ 30.	Orgasm	c.	return to unaroused state
___ 31.	Resolution	d.	orgasmic platform and elevated testes

	Sex Hormones		Sexual Physiology
___ 32.	testosterone	a.	elasticity of vagina
___ 33.	estrogens	b.	ovulation and sperm production
___ 34.	progesterone	c.	corpus luteum and Leydig cell formation
___ 35.	gonadotropin releasing hormone	d.	sex drive
___ 36.	luteinizing hormone	e.	prepares uterus for implantation
___ 37.	follicle stimulating hormone	f.	LH and FSH control

	Menstrual Cycle Phase		Sexual Physiology
___ 38.	follicular	a.	rupture of follicle
___ 39.	ovulatory	b.	increased progesterone and estrogen
___ 40.	luteal	c.	menstruation and proliferation

PART V CLARIFYING YOUR VALUES

The physical changes of the excitement phase are neither constant nor always increasing. Several kinds of distractions can and often do decrease the buildup of sexual tension that characterizes sexual excitement. The following is a list of some possible mental and physical distractions. Rate their effect upon your level of sexual excitement using the scale provided.

	Effect on Sexual Excitement		
Possible Distractions	Decrease	No Change	Increase
Expression of love			
Stomach growling			
Tickling			
Massage			
Honking car horn			
Telephone ringing			
Talking softly (whispers)			
Talking loudly			
Street language (profanity)			
Touching partner's genitals			
Being touched on genitals			
Bright light			
Dimly lit surroundings			
Total darkness			
Hairy body			
Sounds of music			
Unclean body			

Possible Distractions	Effect on Sexual Excitement		
	Decrease	No Change	Increase
Heavy cosmetics			
Constant unchanging caress			
Lack of penile erection			
Lack of vaginal lubrication			
Use of condom			
Use of diaphragm			
Loss of nipple erection			
Full stomach			
Coitus while menstruating			
Sex with person(s) observing			
Worry about school			
Worry about finances			
Other distractions			

PART VI ANSWER KEY TO REVIEW QUIZ

1. True. See text p. 56.
2. False. See text p. 57.
3. True. See text p. 57.
4. True. See text p. 57.
5. True. See text pp. 58-59.
6. False. See text p. 59.
7. True. See text p. 63.
8. False. See text pp. 65-66.
9. True. See text p. 68.
10. False. See text pp. 74-75.
11. (b) See text p. 56.
12. (c) See text p. 56.
13. (d) See text pp. 58-59.
14. (a) See text p. 58.
15. (c) See text pp. 58-59.
16. (b) See text p. 62.
17. (d) See text p. 62.
18. (a) See text p. 63.
19. (c) See text p. 64.
20. (d) See text p. 65.
21. (c) See text p. 65.
22. (c) See text pp. 65-66.
23. (b) See text p. 66.
24. (d) See text p. 66.
25. (b) See text p. 67.
26. (c) See text p. 70.
27. (b) See text p. 78.
28. (b) See text pp. 58-59.
29. (d) See text pp. 62, 65
30. (a) See text p. 65.
31. (c) See text p. 70.
32. (d) See text p. 72.
33. (a) See text p. 72.
34. (e) See text p. 77.
35. (f) See text p. 73.
36. (c) See text p. 73.
37. (b) See text p. 73.
38. (c) See text pp. 75-76.
39. (a) See text p. 76.
40. (b) See text pp. 76-77.

4
Human Reproduction

INTRODUCTION

This chapter continues to explore the biological aspects of human sexuality by examining conception, pregnancy, and childbirth and the problems associated with them. Some of the chapter's main themes involve not only knowledge of, but attitudes toward pregnancy (of both mother and father), prenatal care, sexual activity during pregnancy, childbirth preparation, delivery options, parenting, nursing, birth defects, and infertility.

PART I LEARNING OBJECTIVES

At the conclusion of this chapter, you should be able to:

1. Describe conception by explaining the sequence of events starting with ejaculation and ovulation and ending with implantation.
2. Describe the changes in fetal development during each trimester.
3. Identify the physical, psychological, and social changes that typically occur in the expectant mother and father during each trimester.
4. Explain the need for prenatal care and identify its effects on mother and fetus.
5. List and describe the stages of labor.
6. Define the important terms used in conveying the concepts about human reproduction.
7. Differentiate between hospital delivery and home delivery and discuss the pros and cons of each.
8. Discuss the range of psychological reactions of women toward childbirth and breast feeding.
9. Identify the major types of problem pregnancies; list the most common forms of birth defects; and describe the ways they are detected.
10. State the major causes of infertility in men and women and describe the treatment approaches.

PART II IMPORTANT TERMS AND NAMES TO KNOW

A. Fill in the missing word or words.

1. The release of an egg from an ovary is called __________. (76) — ovulation

2. __________ is the process by which sperm become capable of penetrating an egg. (82) — capacitation

3. The single cell created by the penetration of an egg by a sperm is a(n) __________. (82) — zygote

4. A(n) __________ is a spherical mass of cells with a hollow inner portion containing fluid produced by the cleavage of the fertilized egg. (83) — blastocyst

5. __________ is the attachment of the blastocyst to the lining of the uterus. (83-84) — implantation

6. A(n) __________ __________ is an implantation that occurs outside of the uterus. (84) — ectopic pregnancy

7. A(n) __________ is an unborn child during the first eight weeks after fertilization. (84) — embryo

8. The unborn child from the ninth week after fertilization until birth is called a(n) __________. (84) — fetus

9. A(n) __________ is the organ attached to the wall of the uterus that performs the functions of nutrition, respiration, and excretion for the unborn child. (84) — placenta

10. The inner of the thin sacs of tissue that encloses the developing baby is called the __________. (84) — amnion

11. The __________ __________ is the liquid in which the developing fetus is suspended. (84) — amniotic fluid

12. The __________ __________ is the cylindrical structure connecting the fetus to the placenta. (84) — umbilical cord

13. __________ is swelling due to fluid retention. (88) — edema

14. The settling of the fetal head into position against the pelvic bones is called __________. (89) — engaging

15. __________ __________ represents the combined efforts to insure that the pregnant woman stays healthy and the unborn child has everything needed to grow and develop. (90) — prenatal care

16. The thinning or flattening of the cervix during labor is called __________. (96) — effacement

17. The opening of the mouth of the cervix in preparation for birth is called __________. (96) — dilatation

18. __________ is a hormone made in the posterior pituitary thought to play a role in uterine contractions and lactation stimulation. (96) — oxytocin

19. In childbirth, the appearance of the baby's head at the opening of the vagina is known as __________. (99) — crowning

20. A(n) __________ is an incision in the mother's perineum that gives the baby's head more room to emerge. (99) — episiotomy

21. In childbirth, when the buttocks or feet are the first part of the baby to pass through the opening of the vagina it is called a(n) __________ __________. (99n) — breech presentation

22. __________ is the term used to depict the emotional link partly created by cuddling, cooing, and physical and eye contact by the parent early in the infant's life. (107) — bonding

23. The production of milk by the breasts which usually begins a few days after birth is called __________. (107) — lactation

24. __________ __________ is a chromosome disorder that causes mental retardation and defects of the heart, kidney, and intestine. It is also known as trisomy 21 or mongolism. (109) — Down's syndrome

25. __________ is a procedure used to obtain a sample of amniotic fluid from the uterus of a pregnant woman to analyze for a variety of genetic disorders and biochemical abnormalities in the fetus. (109-110) — amniocentesis

26. A condition in which antibodies from the mother's bloodstream destroy the red blood cells in the fetus, causing anemia, mental retardation, or fetal death is called __________ __________. (111) — Rh incompatibility

27. The inability of a couple to have a baby, usually defined after one year or more of unprotected sexual intercourse without pregnancy is called __________. (111-113) — infertility

B. Match the developer of the delivery method with the style of delivery.

	Developer of Method	Style of Delivery	Key
___	1. Grantly Dick-Reed (102)	a. Birth without violence	Leboyer
___	2. Fernand Lemaze (102-104)	b. Birth without fear	Dick-Reed
___	3. Frederick Leboyer (104)	c. Birth without pain	Lemaze

PART III SELF-TESTING--A PROGRAMMED APPROACH

1. Labor is divided into several stages. The stage which is characterized by the longest duration is the:
   a. First stage (Go to #2)
   b. Second stage (Go to #3)
   c. Third stage (Go to #4)
   d. Fourth stage (Go to #5)

2. The first stage of labor begins with effacement (thinning of the cervix) and dilatation (opening of the mouth of the uterus). When the opening of the cervix reaches 10 centimeters (4 inches), dilatation is complete. This process takes an average of 13 hours. It is by far the longest stage. You are correct. (Go to #6)

3. The second stage of labor lasts about 80 minutes in first pregnancies and about 30 minutes in subsequent ones. Its duration is considered to be moderate; therefore, your answer is incorrect. (Go to #2)

4. The third stage of labor is considered to be the shortest of the three since it lasts about 10 to 12 minutes. It requires only a few minutes following the baby's birth for the placenta to separate from the wall of the uterus and be delivered. Your answer is incorrect. (Go to #2)

5. Although some obstetrics texts define a fourth stage as the time it takes the uterus to contract after delivery of the placenta, it is not commonly considered to be a stage of labor and it is not included in the textbook. The authors describe only three stages: first--lasting about 13 hours; second--lasting 80 minutes for first pregnancies and about 30 minutes in others; and third--taking only 10 to 12 minutes. You are incorrect. (Go to #2)

6. During normal delivery (about 95 percent of the time) the baby's position is in the __________ presentation.
   a. Breech (Go to #7)
   b. Cephalic (Go to #8)
   c. Transverse (Go to #9)
   d. Longitudinal (Go to #10)

7. A Breech Presentation is characterized by the buttocks or feet being delivered first. It occurs in about 4 percent of deliveries. You are incorrect. (Go to #8)

8. A Cephalic Presentation is also known as occiput or vertex presentation. It is characterized by the baby's head being the first part to be delivered. It is the Presentation in 95 percent of deliveries. You are correct. (Go to #11)

9. Transverse Presentations are characterized by the baby lying across the uterus so that a shoulder or arm presents first. This requires turning the baby in delivery or by a cesarean section. These are rare Presentations. You are incorrect. (Go to #8)

10. Longitudinal Presentations may be either cephalic or breech; therefore they are never termed as longitudinal. You are incorrect. (Go to #8)

11. Induced labor is initiated by giving the pregnant woman
    a. HCG (Go to #12)
    b. HMG (Go to #13)
    c. DES (Go to #14)
    d. Oxytocin (Go to #15)

12. HCG is the human chorionic gonadotropin, a hormone secreted by the placenta. It is used as a means to diagnose pregnancy. It cannot induce labor. You are incorrect. (Go to #15)

13. HMG or human menopausal gonadotropin is given in a series of injections because it acts on the ovaries and will induce ovulation. It is used to treat women who do not ovulate, but usually only after clomiphene has been tried. It therefore has no effect upon labor. You are incorrect. (Go to #15)

14. DES is an artificial estrogen which was used on pregnant women who were prone to spontaneous abortion. It is also used as the "morning after pill." If given in large doses it can interfere with the implantation of a fertilized ovum in the uterus. It is not a recommended form of contraception and is never used to induce labor. You are incorrect. (Go to #15)

15. Oxytocin is a pituitary hormone believed to be involved in the onset of labor. It is usually the drug used for inducing labor. You are correct. (Go to #16)

16. Down's Syndrome is a chromosome disorder which causes severe mental retardation and defects of the heart, kidneys, and intestines. Its incidence increases with
    a. maternal infection with German measles (Go to #17)
    b. prematurity (Go to #18)
    c. advanced age of the mother (Go to #19)
    d. Rh incompatibility (Go to #20)

17. German measles (rubella) does produce birth defects including deafness, cataracts, heart defects, mental retardation, and retarded growth, but does not result in Down's Syndrome. You are incorrect. (Go to #19)

18. Prematurity results in health problems (respiratory, seizures, and infections) and is a leading cause of newborn death. Premature births are associated with maternal illness, malfunction of the placenta, smoking, and youthful (teenage) pregnancies. It does not, however, result in Down's Syndrome. You are incorrect. (Go to #19)

19. Down's Syndrome is a chromosome disorder whose incidence increases with advanced maternal age. You are correct.

20. Rh incompatibility is caused by antibodies from the mother's bloodstream destroying the red blood cells in the fetus causing anemia, mental retardation, or death in the baby. This only occurs when the mother's blood does not have the Rh factor (Rh negative) and the fetus does have the Rh factor (Rh positive). This risk is slight in a first pregnancy but increases with subsequent ones. It can be prevented by medication. It does not cause the chromosomal disorder Down's Syndrome (trisomy 21 or mongolism). You are incorrect. (Go to #19)

PART IV REVIEW QUIZ

A. True or False

___ 1. Sperm can retain their capacity to penetrate the egg for 36 hours.

___ 2. After a year of unprotected coitus, pregnancy occurs in about 8 out of 10 couples.

___ 3. The collection of cells which implants into the lining of the uterus is called a morula.

___ 4. Average pregnancies last about 266 days.

___ 5. Before the sixth week, male and female embryos are anatomically indistinguishable.

___ 6. Missing a menstrual period is a certain sign of pregnancy.

___ 7. Babies born in the second trimester of pregnancy have a poor chance of survival.

___ 8. Almost every drug a pregnant woman uses will cross the placenta and enter the circulation of the fetus.

___ 9. A sustained drop in the fetal heart rate may indicate fetal distress.

___ 10. Most birth defects are inherited.

___ 11. Women who do not ovulate may be helped by a pill which induces ovulation called clomiphene.

___ 12. Men with low sperm counts are advised to ejaculate daily in order to increase sperm counts.

B. Multiple Choice--Select the Best Answer

___ 13. Fertilization of the egg usually occurs in the
a. vagina
b. uterus
c. Fallopian tubes
d. ovaries

___ 14. The attachment of the blastocyst to the lining of the uterus is a process known as
a. transudation
b. implantation
c. burrowing
d. impregnation

___ 15. Ectopic pregnancies can occur
a. in the Fallopian tubes
b. in the abdomen
c. in the uterus
d. a and b above

___ 16. The average pregnancy lasts for
a. 9 months
b. 270 days
c. 266 days
d. a and b above

___ 17. The events of pregnancy are usually broken down into periods known as
a. semesters
b. trimesters
c. prenatal stages
d. none of the above

___ 18. Recognizable male and female genitalia appear in the
a. first month of pregnancy
b. second month of pregnancy
c. third month of pregnancy
d. fourth month of pregnancy

___ 19. All of the major organs are formed in the developing baby by the beginning of the
a. third month
b. fourth month
c. fifth month
d. sixth month

___ 20. The most accurate and widely available test for pregnancy two weeks after a missed period is
a. testing woman's urine in laboratory animals
b. the rabbit test
c. the beta-subunit HCG radioimmunoassay
d. immunological tests detecting presence of HCG in woman's urine

___ 21. The average full-term baby weighs about _____ lbs and is about _____ inches long.
a. 7, 20
b. 6, 18
c. 5½, 17
d. 8, 21

___ 22. Malnourished babies are often
a. born with low birth weight
b. born prematurely
c. born with brain damage and retardation
d. all of the above

___ 23. Fetal heart defects have been reported in pregnant mothers who use
a. birth control pills
b. librium
c. equanil
d. all of the above

___ 24. Electronic equipment is often used to check the progress of the fetus during delivery. The technique is called
a. fetal telegraphy
b. electrofetography
c. fetal monitoring
d. none of the above

___ 25. The two major causes of female infertility are
a. failure to ovulate and blockage of the Fallopian tubes
b. abnormal cervical mucus and blocked Fallopian tubes
c. birth defects of the reproductive organs and tumors
d. infections and allergy to sperm

C. Matching

Pregnancy Period	Fetal Development
___ 26. First trimester	a. major organs are formed
___ 27. Second trimester	b. fatty tissue deposits
___ 28. Third trimester	c. fetal movement and activity

Drug Usage	Effects on Fetus
___ 29. smoking tobacco	a. lower birth weight
___ 30. beverage alcohol	b. cleft palate
___ 31. aspirin	c. masculinization of female
___ 32. valium	d. cancer of the vagina
___ 33. testosterone	e. fetal bleeding
___ 34. estrogens	f. convulsions and depressed breathing
___ 35. diethylstilbestrol	g. uncertain in humans
___ 36. heroin	h. improper formation of penis
___ 37. marijuana	i. facial and eye abnormalities

PART V CLARIFYING YOUR VALUES

If you had the ability to award large sums of money for research on reproduction, rank order the priorities you would use for funding research proposals. Include your major reason for assigning each rank.

Research Proposal	Rank	Reason
Test tube babies		
Birth defects		
Miscarriages		
Prenatal nutrition		
Addicted babies		
Prematurity		
Ectopic pregnancy		
Infertility		

PART VI ANSWERS TO REVIEW QUIZ

1. True. See text p. 81.
2. True. See text pp. 81-82.
3. False. See text p. 83.
4. True. See text p. 84.
5. True. See text p. 85.
6. False. See text p. 86.
7. True. See text p. 87.
8. True. See text p. 92.
9. True. See text p. 100.
10. False. See text p. 109.
11. True. See text p. 113.
12. False. See text p. 113.
13. (c) See text p. 82.
14. (b) See text pp. 83-84.
15. (d) See text p. 84.
16. (c) See text p. 84.
17. (b) See text p. 84.
18. (c) See text p. 85.
19. (b) See text p. 87.
20. (d) See text p. 86.
21. (a) See text p. 88.
22. (d) See text p. 90.
23. (d) See text p. 93.
24. (c) See text p. 100.
25. (a) See text p. 111.
26. (a) See text pp. 84-85.
27. (c) See text p. 87.
28. (b) See text p. 88.
29. (a) See text pp. 92-93.
30. (i) See text p. 94.
31. (e) See text p. 92.
32. (b) See text p. 92.
33. (c) See text p. 92.
34. (h) See text p. 92.
35. (d) See text p. 92.
36. (f) See text p. 92.
37. (g) See text p. 94.

5
Contraception

INTRODUCTION

Chapter Five examines the currently available methods of birth control and the future trends in contraception. It includes the reasons for using birth control, the various methods used, how each method works, how well each one works, the health risks, and the effects on sexuality. It also reviews the options available if pregnancy occurs, the psychology of contraceptive use, and research that is underway to improve the range of choices available.

PART I LEARNING OBJECTIVES

At the conclusion of this chapter, you should be able to:

1. List the factors which affect an individual's or couple's decisions about birth control.
2. Discuss the major reasons for using birth control.
3. Describe the factors that complicate our ability to evaluate the effectiveness and safety of contraceptive methods.
4. Differentiate between theoretical effectiveness and actual effectiveness of a particular birth control method.
5. Identify the commonly used methods of contraception, discuss the use, effectiveness, side-effects, safety, and sexual effects of each method.
6. List the surgical procedures used to prevent pregnancy; describe each procedure; and discuss the degree of difficulty and safety in each procedure.
7. Explain the post-conception methods of birth control and the controversy surrounding each method.
8. Discuss why some people who don't want a pregnancy avoid the use of contraception or misuse the method of birth control they have selected.
9. Contrast the desire to avoid pregnancy with the desire to delay the timing of pregnancy in terms of choice and consistency of use of contraceptive method.
10. Describe the future trends in male and female contraception and explain how these new directions are being pursued.

PART II IMPORTANT TERMS TO KNOW

Fill in the missing word or words.

1. A(n) __________ pill is a birth control pill containing a synthetic estrogen and a progesterone-like substance. (122) — combination

2. A(n) __________ is a contraceptive pill containing only progesterone in low dosage. (122) — minipill

3. A(n) __________ pill was an earlier type of birth control pill that was banned because it was found to cause cancer of the uterus. (124n) — sequential

4. __________ is one of the side-effects of contraceptive pill use and it is characterized by brown pigment spots on the face. (124) — chloasma

5. The formation of a blood clot in a vein causing inflammation and swelling with the possibility that the clot may break off and cause serious damage in the lungs or brain is called a __________ disease. (125) — thromboembolic

6. A(n) __________ __________ is a small plastic object that is inserted into the uterus through the vagina and cervix. (127) — intrauterine device (IUD)

7. A(n) __________ is a round, shallow dome of thin rubber stretched over a flexible ring and inserted into the vagina to act as a mechanical barrier that blocks the mouth of the cervix. (131) — diaphragm

8. A(n) __________ __________ fits snugly over the cervix and functions as a mechanical barrier that blocks the mouth of the cervix. (131) — cervical cap

9.	A(n) __________ is a thin sheath of latex rubber or tissue from a lamb's intestine that fits snugly over the penis. (132)	condom
10.	Chemical contraceptives that come in varieties including foams, jellies, creams, and tablets or suppositories are known as __________. (134)	spermicides
11.	The __________ __________ of birth control is a technique of determining the days in the menstrual cycle when the risk of pregnancy is low. It is a form of the rhythm method. (135)	calendar method
12.	The __________ __________ of birth control involves daily recording of the basal body temperature to pinpoint the time of ovulation. (137)	temperature method
13.	The __________ __________ of birth control depends on changes in the cervical mucus which are thought to indicate the time of ovulation. (137)	ovulation method
14.	__________ involves the removal of the penis from the vagina before ejaculation occurs. (141)	withdrawal
15.	Using a liquid to flush the vagina is called __________. (141)	douching
16.	Voluntarily not engaging in sexual intercourse is known as __________. (141)	abstention
17.	A surgical procedure done on either men or women to prevent union of sperm and egg is called __________. (137)	sterilization
18.	A(n) __________ __________ is a procedure involving literally tying the Fallopian tubes. (138)	tubal ligation

19. A(n) __________ is an operation involving an incision through the abdominal wall infrequently used for sterilization. (139) — laparotomy

20. A(n) __________ is the surgical removal (total or partial) of the uterus. (139) — hysterectomy

21. A(n) __________ is the surgical removal of the ovaries. (139) — ovariectomy

22. A(n) __________ is the surgical procedure for the sterilization of the male consisting of cutting and tying each vas deferens. (139) — vasectomy

23. ___ ___ ___ is the acronym for a high dose of estrogen given to prevent implantation and provide a form of "after the fact" birth control--known as the "Morning After Pill." (141) — DES

24. __________ __________ is a technique to draw out the endometrial lining of the uterus by inserting a thin, flexible plastic tube through the cervix and applying suction by a syringe or pump. (141-142) — menstrual extraction

25. __________ is the termination of a pregnancy before the fetus can survive outside the uterus. __________ __________ occur naturally due to medical problems; __________ __________ are done intentionally. (142) — abortion; spontaneous abortions; induced abortions

26. __________ __________ is a method usually chosen during the first trimester of pregnancy which involves dilating the cervix, placing a small plastic tube into the uterus and connecting it to an electric pump which removes fetal tissue, placenta, and other membranes from the uterus by suction. (142) — vacuum aspiration

27. __________ __________ abortions are done by injecting prostaglandins into the amniotic sac, dripping them slowly into a vein, or placing them in the vagina. (142) — prostaglandin induced

28. __________ __________ abortions are done by injecting 7 oz. of salt solution into the amniotic sac after an equal amount of amniotic fluid has been removed. (142) — saline induced

29. __________ and __________ is a process involving dilating the cervix and gently scraping the lining of the uterus with a metal instrument. (143) — dilatation curettage

30. A(n) __________ is an incision of the uterus that can be used during the second trimester for an abortion. (143) — hysterotomy

PART III SELF-TESTING--A PROGRAMMED APPROACH

1. The main reason for using birth control is to
   a. space pregnancies (Go to #2)
   b. prevent an unwanted pregnancy (Go to #3)
   c. avoid potential genetic disorders (Go to #4)
   d. limit family size (Go to #5)

2. Spacing pregnancies is certainly a good reason to use birth control, especially when one considers the economic drain on the family and the health of the mother when pregnancies are too close together. However, this is not the main reason for birth control, as it is too narrowly focused. It includes primarily only those who have been previously pregnant. You are incorrect. (Go to #3)

3. Unwanted pregnancies can cause emotional turmoil, health risks, and financial burdens. The main reason for using birth control is to prevent an unwanted pregnancy regardless of one's age, marital status, or family situation. You are correct. (Go to #6)

4. Genetic disorders can be avoided by using a birth control method as can the birth defects associated with them. This is more likely to be an idiosyncratic rather than a common or generally applied reason. Your answer is incorrect. (Go to #3)

5. Limiting family size is a fairly common reason people give for practicing birth control, but it is mostly limited to married couples or those who already have children. It is too specific. You are incorrect. (Go to #3)

6. When evaluating the effectiveness or safety of a contraceptive, we can confidently accept information from which of the following sources?
   a. Media--newspaper, TV, or radio news reports (Go to #7)
   b. Research articles (Go to #8)
   c. Scientific studies (Go to #9)
   d. None of the above (Go to #10)

7. In their eagerness to report the latest "news" about the "breakthroughs" in contraception in a condensed format, the media often oversimplifies, misinterprets, or draws unwarranted conclusions about the method. Be aware as well that much of the media is sponsored by drug company advertising. You are incorrect. (Go to #10)

8. Research articles, even those in professionally peer-reviewed journals, can have a built-in bias as much of the research they describe is financed by the drug companies that manufacture the contraceptive. They have an obvious interest in presenting the research in a manner which will not impugn their merchandise. You are incorrect. (Go to #10)

9. Scientific studies, even those free of the "bias" of drug company funding, are not necessarily generalizable to you as an individual. Studies conducted on subjects who are more equivalent to you (i.e., same age, socioeconomic status, educational level, cultural background, etc.) are more meaningful to you than studies which were done using other groups. However, there are often wide differences in the frequency of side-effects reported by different investigators that can be attributed to differences in research designs, control groups, and methods used to gather and analyze data. You are incorrect. (Go to #10)

10. You are correct. Each of the sources has serious limitations. Scientific studies come closer to being the most valid source if they involved subjects close to your age, cultural background, educational level, and socioeconomic status. However, their findings must always be examined in light of one's own personal situation; for example, are the side-effects reported more or less serious for YOU than the risks of pregnancy and childbirth? How important is it for YOU to avoid pregnancy? (Go to #11)

11. Considering the methods of contraception that are available to most American men and women today, which methods have an excellent effectiveness rating?
    a. Combination birth control pill, condom and diaphragm (used together), IUD, condom and foam (used together). (Go to #12)
    b. Combination birth control pill, diaphragm and jelly (used together), IUD, vasectomy (Go to #13)
    c. Combination birth control pill, IUD, tubal ligation, spermicide (Go to #14)
    d. Combination birth control pill, IUD, vasectomy, cervical cap (Go to #15)

12. All of the methods included in this response choice have an effectiveness rating of "excellent" with an ideal failure rate of 1 percent or less. You are correct. (Go to #16)

13. Diaphragm and jelly have an ideal failure rate of 3 percent with an effectiveness rating of "very good." Although all other methods were rated as excellent, the inclusion of diaphragm and jelly makes this an incorrect answer. (Go to #12)

14. Spermicides used alone without another method of birth control (e.g., condom) have only a "good" effectiveness rating. Although all other methods were rated as excellent, the inclusion of spermicide makes this an incorrect answer. (Go to #12)

15. The cervical cap is a device similar to the diaphragm. It is currently experiencing an increase in use in the United States. It seems to have a slightly improved effectiveness over the diaphragm. Its effectiveness rating is at the "very good" level and its ideal failure rate is 2 percent. Although all other methods were rated as excellent, the inclusion of the cervical cap makes this an incorrect answer. (Go to #12)

16. Since there is general agreement that the currently available contraceptive methods leave something to be desired, research is underway to improve the range of choices. The most intense interest is presently focused on which of the following approaches?
    a. Using ultrasound to produce temporary sterility by blocking sperm production (Go to #17)
    b. Developing an anti-pregnancy vaccine (Go to #18)
    c. Developing a male birth control pill (Go to #19)
    d. Testing MPA, a long-acting contraceptive (Go to #20)

17. The use of ultrasound is extremely new and experimental. It is not being investigated with much vigor at this point in time. You are incorrect. (Go to #19)

18. An anti-pregnancy vaccine is of much interest in the scientific community because it is one of the most promising approaches in female contraception. There is some concern that the women's movement has made both men and women look with some suspicion on female-oriented contraception. Therefore, greater efforts seem to be focused on finding a male alternative. You are incorrect. (Go to #19)

19. Intense interest focuses on the possibility of developing a male birth control pill. Several reasons are obvious (e.g., women ovulate once a month, men produce sperm cells in the millions each day; women have been the guinea pigs for too long; etc.). Clinical trials have not yet found a pill without undesirable side-effects so research efforts have been rekindled. You are correct.

20. MPA, medroxyprogesterone acetate, is being used as a long-acting contraceptive in other countries but its effectiveness is no better than the combination birth control pill. It has been recently reported that MPA may cause cancer of the uterus, and it is not being energetically pursued or financed. You are incorrect. (Go to #19)

PART IV REVIEW QUIZ

A. True or False

___ 1. A landmark study of teenage pregnancy conducted in 1979 revealed that half of all unwed teenage pregnancies occurred in girls who never used any birth control method.

___ 2. The best contraceptive method based on effectiveness and safety is the birth control pill.

___ 3. The actual effectiveness of a contraceptive method is usually higher than the theoretical effectiveness.

___ 4. The longer a person uses a particular birth control method, the less effective it becomes.

___ 5. Insertion of an IUD is usually done just following a menstrual period.

___ 6. The calendar method is the least reliable among the rhythm methods of contraception.

___ 7. Laparotomy is the most frequently performed procedure for female sterilization.

___ 8. A vasectomy is the simplest and safest form of surgical contraception.

___ 9. The abortion method used depends upon the age of the pregnant woman.

___ 10. Modern abortion techniques are less risky to the mother than a full term pregnancy.

B. Multiple Choice--Select the Best Answer

___ 11. Health risks during pregnancy are highest in women of which age(s)?
a. under 18
b. over 35
c. between 28 and 34
d. a and b above

___ 12. How many of the one million teenagers who become pregnant in the U.S. each year obtain abortions?
a. 500,000
b. 400,000
c. 300,000
d. 200,000

____ 13. An unwanted pregnancy can
  a. disrupt career plans
  b. create financial burdens
  c. create later sexual problems
  d. all of the above

____ 14. Actual effectiveness of a particular contraceptive method is due to
  a. method failure
  b. user failure
  c. a and b above
  d. none of the above

____ 15. The birth control pills which were banned were found to cause cancer of the uterus. The type that were banned contained
  a. a combination of synthetic estrogen and progesterone
  b. only estrogen in the first 15 pills and only progesterone in the others
  c. progesterone only in low dosage
  d. a and c above

____ 16. The most serious risk to women using birth control pills involve(s)
  a. malignancies
  b. disorders of the circulatory system
  c. alterations in liver functions
  d. increased susceptibility to vaginal infections

____ 17. The exact way an IUD works is
  a. unknown
  b. by interfering with ovulation
  c. by reducing cilia movement in the Fallopian tubes
  d. by interfering with implantation

____ 18. Insertion of an IUD is usually done
  a. during a menstrual period
  b. during a 5-day period prior to an expected menstruation
  c. immediately following the menstrual period
  d. anytime during the month

____ 19. Expulsion rates of IUDs are highest
  a. in young women
  b. in women who have had no children
  c. during menstruation
  d. all of the above

____ 20. In order to increase the effectiveness of the diaphragm it should be
  a. used with a spermicide
  b. used with a condom
  c. left in for at least 6 hours
  d. all of the above

___ 21. A condom used alone is about as effective as
- a. a diaphragm and spermicide
- b. the rhythm method
- c. a cervical cap and spermicide
- d. the minipill

___ 22. Spermicides work by
- a. killing sperm
- b. providing a mechanical barrier to sperm
- c. increasing the pH of the vagina
- d. a and b above

___ 23. The most effective of the rhythm methods is
- a. calendar method
- b. temperature method
- c. ovulation method
- d. none of the methods is considered to be effective

___ 24. A man and his sexual partner should use another form of birth control after he has had a vasectomy until
- a. 6 weeks have passed since the surgery
- b. at least two consecutive semen tests show no sperm
- c. 8 weeks have passed since the vasectomy
- d. the semen test shows no live sperm in the ejaculate

___ 25. The most effective method of contraception is
- a. birth control pills
- b. tubal ligation
- c. vasectomy
- d. MPA

C. Matching--Match the abortion method with the length of pregnancy.

Abortion Method	Length of Pregnancy*
___ 26. Menstrual extraction	a. First trimester
___ 27. Vacuum aspiration	b. After the 14th week
___ 28. Prostaglandin-induced	c. Not typically viewed as an abortion; however, is performed when a period is expected and up to 2 weeks following
___ 29. Saline-induced	
___ 30. D & C	d. 15 weeks after last menstrual period
___ 31. Hysterotomy	

*An answer may be used more than once.

PART V CLARIFYING YOUR VALUES

Choosing a contraceptive method involves considering many factors. There is no one contraceptive method that is always the best and the safest. Some are more appropriate than others depending on age, history of pregnancy, amount of sexual activity, medical conditions, etc. Once you have all the facts about the methods, how do you really decide?

The chances are that you decide about contraception pretty much the way you decide about other health behaviors; that is, based upon your beliefs. You're probably like most of us who allow our feelings and emotions to modify our beliefs which, in turn, affects our actions.

One way to evaluate the process used in making decisions is to examine our beliefs or to clarify our values about an issue--in this case--contraception. List the contraceptive method that you currently use or think you would use if you are not currently using any contraceptive method (if you are sexually active). If you are not sexually active, list the contraceptive method you think you would use if you became sexually active. Circle the response which most closely indicates the way you feel about each reason for using the method.

SA = Strongly Agree
AS = Agree Somewhat
UN = Undecided
DS = Disagree Somewhat
SD = Strongly Disagree

CONTRACEPTIVE METHOD ________________________

	Reason for Decision	Feeling About Reason				
1.	It's the most effective	SA	AS	UN	DS	SD
2.	It's the safest	SA	AS	UN	DS	SD
3.	It's the least expensive	SA	AS	UN	DS	SD
4.	It's the most convenient	SA	AS	UN	DS	SD
5.	It's what my partner wants	SA	AS	UN	DS	SD
6.	It's what most of my peers use	SA	AS	UN	DS	SD
7.	It's compatible with my lifestyle	SA	AS	UN	DS	SD
8.	It's compatible with my religious views	SA	AS	UN	DS	SD
9.	It's compatible with my personality	SA	AS	UN	DS	SD
10.	It's what I'm pressured into using	SA	AS	UN	DS	SD

Scoring

Reasons 1, 2, 3, 4, and 8 are scored +2 for SA, +1 for AS, 0 for UN, -1 for DS, and -2 for SD. Subtotal A = ________

Reasons 5, 6, 7, 9, and 10 are scored -2 for SA, -1 for AS, 0 for UN, +1 for DS, and +2 for SD. Subtotal B = ________

A + B = ________

Evaluation

If your total of A+B is positive (e.g., +1 to +20) your decision was based more on information than emotions. If the total was negative your decision was based more on emotions.

PART VI ANSWERS TO REVIEW QUIZ

1. True. See text p. 119.
2. False. See text p. 121.
3. False. See text pp. 121-122.
4. False. See text p. 122.
5. False. See text p. 127.
6. True. See text p. 137.
7. False. See text p. 139.
8. True. See text p. 139.
9. False. See text p. 142.
10. True. See text pp. 143-144.
11. (d) See text p. 120.
12. (c) See text p. 120.
13. (d) See text pp. 120-121.
14. (c) See text p. 122.
15. (b) See text p. 124.
16. (b) See text p. 124.
17. (a) See text p. 127.
18. (a) See text p. 127.
19. (d) See text p. 128.
20. (d) See text p. 131.
21. (a) See text p. 134.
22. (d) See text p. 135.
23. (c) See text p. 137.
24. (b) See text p. 139.
25. (b) See text p. 150.
26. (c) See text pp. 141-142.
27. (a) See text p. 142.
28. (b) See text p. 142.
29. (b) See text p. 142.
30. (d) See text p. 143.
31. (b) See text p. 143.

6

Developmental Sexuality: A Biological View

INTRODUCTION

This chapter considers developmental sexuality in each stage of the life cycle from a biological viewpoint. It includes the biological aspects of human development during the prenatal period, infancy, childhood, puberty, and during the process of aging.

PART I LEARNING OBJECTIVES

At the conclusion of this chapter, you should be able to:

1. Identify the genetic and hormonal mechanisms that control prenatal sexual differentiation.
2. Describe the development of the external genitals from the embryonic tissues in male and female fetuses.
3. Explain the process of male and female brain differentiation and identify the differences.
4. Identify the causes of abnormal prenatal development and explain each cause including chromosomal, genetic, and hormonal or drug exposures.
5. Discuss the biologic developmental sexuality of infancy and childhood and contrast the range of physical sexual responsiveness between boys and girls.
6. Describe the hormonal control of puberty and the physical changes which occur in both males and females during adolescence and discuss the relationship between pubertal hormones and sexual behavior.
7. Describe the changing sexuality of later adult life and contrast the differences in male and female patterns of reproductive aging.
8. Discuss the argument among scientists about the relative importance of nature verses nurture in controlling or modifying human sexual development.
9. Explain why a girl's reaction to menarche may be a negative one and why a shift in attitude during the past two decades may be occurring about menstruation; and describe the relationship between toxic shock syndrome and the use of tampons.
10. Explain the physiologic and psychologic basis for nocturnal emissions.

PART II IMPORTANT TERMS TO KNOW

1.	The time from conception to birth is called the __________ period. (152)	prenatal
2.	__________ __________ is the process that begins at the moment of conception to create a normal male or female. (152)	sexual differentiation
3.	The substance that controls the transformation of the primitive gonads into testes in the embryo is __________ __________. (153)	H-Y antigen
4.	The __________ __________ __________ substance is a chemical secreted by the embryonic testes which causes the Mullerian duct system to shrink and practically disappear. (153)	Mullerian duct inhibiting
5.	__________ is a hormone similar to testosterone which stimulates embryonic development of the penis, scrotum, and prostate gland. (153)	dihydrotestosterone
6.	Hormones that develop and maintain male secondary sex characteristics in males and, if in large quantities, promote masculinization in females are called __________. (153)	androgens
7.	The __________ __________ is the passage through which the testes migrate down into the scrotum during the eighth or ninth month of fetal development. (155)	inguinal canal
8.	__________ __________ is a sex chromosome abnormality marked by an extra X chromosome in a genetic male giving a 47, XXY pattern. (156)	Klinefelter's syndrome

9. __________ __________ is a sex chromosome abnormality caused by a missing chromosome giving a 45, X pattern. (157) — Turner's syndrome

10. A person with both testicular and ovarian tissue is a(n) __________ __________. (158) — true hermaphrodite

11. A(n) __________ is a person born with gonads matching the sex chromosomes but with a genital appearance that resembles the opposite sex. (158) — pseudo-hermaphrodite

12. The __________ __________ is an inherited disorder involving an enzyme block in the adrenal glands in which excessive amounts of androgens are produced during fetal development causing females to have masculinized genitals. (158) — androgenital syndrome

13. The __________ __________ __________ is an inherited condition in which tissues are insensitive to the effects of testosterone and a chromosomal male 46, XY develops female genitals. (159) — testicular feminization syndrome

14. Undescended testes are called __________. (162) — cryptorchid

15. The onset of menstruation is called __________. (162) — menarche

16. The period of fast bone growth usually occurring in the early or middle teens which is caused by the rising sex hormone levels of puberty is called the __________ __________ __________. (162-163) — adolescent growth spurt

17. __________ is the period during which menstruation generally stops in women in their late forties or fifties. (170) — menopause

18. The __________ __________ is a condition which occurs in about 5 percent of men over 60 years of age and is sometimes compared to menopause in women. (170) — male climacteric

19. __________ __________ __________ is a rare but serious condition that is believed to be related to the use of tampons. (168) — toxic shock syndrome

20. __________ __________ is the ejaculation which often occurs in young males during the sleep cycle and is thought to provide a physiological means of release of accumulated sexual tension. (171) — nocturnal emission

PART III SELF-TESTING--A PROGRAMMED APPROACH

1. At the time of fertilization, the genetic codes for male and female sexual differentiation are set in place. However, if a chemical substance is not present, the primitive gonads will not differentiate, rather
   a. they will develop into ovaries (Go to #2)
   b. they will develop into testes (Go to #3)
   c. a true hermaphrodite will develop (Go to #4)
   d. a pseudohermaphrodite will develop (Go to #5)

2. A chemical substance, H-Y antigen, which is controlled by the Y chromosome, is necessary to start the transformation of the primitive gonads into testes. If it is not present, the primitive gonads will always develop into ovaries. You are correct. (Go to #6)

3. In order for testes to develop, a chemical substance called H-Y antigen, which is controlled by the Y chromosome, must be present in order for the primitive gonads to be transformed into testes. If there is no H-Y antigen present, the primitive gonads will always develop into ovaries regardless of the genetic code. You are incorrect. (Go to #2)

4. A true hermaphrodite is a person born with both testicular and ovarian tissues. The chemical substance necessary for sexual differentiation, H-Y antigen, was present but the differentiation was not unilateral. You are incorrect. (Go to #2)

5. Pseudohermaphrodites are usually the result of inherited conditions in which androgen production is altered. The two types of chromosomal males who exhibit pseudohermaphroditism have the H-Y antigen present; the chromosomal female who exhibits pseudohermaphroditism would not require it in the first place. You are incorrect. (Go to #2)

6. Two of the most common chromosome abnormalities are Klinefelter's syndrome and Turner's syndrome. Klinefelter's is the more common of the two occurring about once in every 500 male births and is due to the male receiving an extra X chromosome. As a result
   a. sperm production is reduced (Go to #7)
   b. testosterone production is reduced (Go to #8)
   c. external genitalia are feminized (Go to #9)
   d. internal sex structures are altered so that the prostate is missing (Go to #10)

7. Sperm production is not only reduced but the structure of the testes has been so dramatically altered that no sperm production occurs. You are incorrect. (Go to #8)

8. Testosterone production is usually reduced. This may explain why males with Klinefelter's syndrome usually have low sexual drive and impotency. They also exhibit passivity and have relatively low ambition, which may be related to their testosterone deficiency. You are correct. (Go to #11)

9. There is no feminization of the external genitalia. Although men with Klinefelter's syndrome may have poor muscular development and enlarged breasts, their penis and scrotum appear normal. However, the microscopic structure of their testes is abnormal and may account for the fact that no sperm production occurs. You are incorrect. (Go to #8)

10. There is no apparent alteration of the internal sex structures and the prostate is intact. Males with Klinefelter's syndrome are, however, sterile. You are incorrect. (Go to #8)

11. The minor hormonal differences between girls and boys during childhood are caused by the hormonal activity of the
    a. hypothalamus (Go to #12)
    b. pituitary (Go to #13)
    c. adrenals (Go to #14)
    d. gonads (Go to #15)

12. The hypothalamus does not start to signal (i.e., it does not produce the pituitary releasing factors that initiate pituitary gonadotropin secretions) the pituitary until puberty. You are incorrect. (Go to #14)

13. The pituitary gland does not begin producing sizable amounts of gonadotropins until the hypothalamus signals it by the secretion of pituitary releasing factors. This does not occur until puberty. The pituitary gland is, sexually speaking, inactive. You are incorrect. (Go to #14)

14. In childhood, there are few hormonal differences between girls and boys. This is due to the fact that the hypothalamus, pituitary, and gonads are relatively inactive (sexually) until puberty. The major source of both testosterone and estrogen in childhood is the adrenal glands. Since the adrenals are essentially identical in both sexes, the sex hormone production is very similar. You are correct. (Go to #16)

15. The gonads, the major source of sex hormone production during adolescence, are relatively nonfunctional during childhood. You are incorrect. (Go to #14)

16. The average age of menarche has been constantly decreasing during the last century on a decade-by-decade basis. Several factors have been related to the decrease including socioeconomic status, climate, heredity, family size, and nutrition. Recent research seems to suggest that as one of these factors has become more uniform, the decrease has begun to level off. Which one of these factors has been linked to the decrease in age of menarche?
   a. socioeconomic status (Go to #17)
   b. climate (Go to #18)
   c. heredity (Go to #19)
   d. nutrition (Go to #20)

17. There have been little variations in the difference between SES levels of Americans in the past 25 years. All levels have experienced an increase but there is some evidence that the difference has widened rather than decreased. SES has not become more uniform. You are incorrect. (Go to #20)

18. Climate changes very slowly. The earth has increased its temperature ever so gradually during the past several hundred years. Climate has not changed radically enough during one decade to account for the dramatic reduction in age of menarche. You are incorrect. (Go to #20)

19. Genetic makeup tends to be less uniform today than it was 100 years ago. this may be due in some part to the relaxation of social, cultural, and religious bans against intergroup marriages. The increase in population mobility, industrialization, and urbanization have had some effect. There are more intergroup marriages today than 100 years ago, broadening the genetic makeup of individuals, especially in the U.S. Our heredity is less uniform than it was and continues to diversify decade-by-decade. You are incorrect. (Go to #20)

20. There is some scientific evidence that appears to support the idea that we have a reduction in the differences between nutritional levels among people in the U.S. The increase in this uniformity has been reported to correlate significantly with the leveling off in age of menarche. The influence of nutrition on menstruation was also demonstrated in a study which found a statistically significant negative correlation between the percentage of body fat and age of menarche. Another study showed a statistically significant correlation between female long-distance runners and ballet dancers in training and menstruation. You are correct.

PART IV REVIEW QUIZ

<u>A. True or False</u>

___ 1. Prenatal sexual differentiation is largely controlled by genetic and hormonal mechanisms.

___ 2. Female sexual differentiation does not depend on hormones.

___ 3. By the 8th week of development, there is a clear difference in the internal sex structure of a male and female fetus.

___ 4. Pseudohermaphroditism is caused by a chromosome disorder.

___ 5. The major difference in hormonal output between males and females occurs during puberty.

___ 6. The adolescent growth spurt typically occurs two years earlier in females than in males.

___ 7. There is a relationship between age of pubescence and amount and start of sexual activity (e.g., late maturers have less and later teenage sexual activity than early maturers).

___ 8. The timing of menopause and the symptoms that accompany it are quite similar among women (e.g., hot flashes, irritability, thinning of breasts and genitals, etc.).

___ 9. A majority of men over the age of 60 years will experience the male climacteric.

___ 10. Prostate problems in men seem to increase with age.

B. Multiple Choice--Select the Best Answer

___ 11. Sexual differentiation starts from the moment of conception and is largely controlled by
a. chromosomes
b. hormones
c. a combination of genetic and hormonal mechanisms
d. prevalence of embryonic duct systems

___ 12. The chemical substance H-Y antigen is controlled by the
a. hypothalamus
b. pituitary
c. X chromosome
d. Y chromosome

___ 13. Male internal sex structures develop from the
a. Mullerian duct system
b. Wolffian duct system
c. interstitial tissue
d. adrenogenital tissue

___ 14. At which week of development is there a clear difference in the internal sex structure of a male and female fetus?
a. 8th week
b. 10th week
c. 12th week
d. 14th week

___ 15. The genital tubercle will develop into
  a. the shaft of the penis in the male
  b. the perineum in both sexes
  c. the clitoris in the female
  d. the labia in the female and the scrotum in the male

___ 16. The best-documented structural differences between male and female brains are in the
  a. hypothalamus
  b. cerebral cortex
  c. cerebellum
  d. pituitary

___ 17. When a genetic male has an extra X chromosome, it results in a condition known as
  a. Klinefelter's syndrome
  b. Turner's syndrome
  c. adrenogenital syndrome
  d. testicular feminization syndrome

___ 18. When a genetic female has one X chromosome missing, it results in a condition known as
  a. Klinefelter's syndrome
  b. Turner's syndrome
  c. adrenogenital syndrome
  d. testicular feminization syndrome

___ 19. A true hermaphrodite has
  a. one ovary and one testis
  b. gonads which are mixtures of ovarian and testicular tissue
  c. both a and b above
  d. none of the above

___ 20. Adrenogenital syndrome females
  a. have female genitals
  b. have female internal sex structures
  c. are infertile
  d. none of the above

___ 21. Testicular feminization syndrome is an inherited condition in which
  a. estrogens alter the function of the testes
  b. testosterone and other androgens have no effect on body tissues
  c. a clitoris, labia, and vagina develop
  d. both b and c above

___ 22. Prolonged positioning of one or both testes in the abdomen
  a. creates an increased risk of cancer
  b. damage their sperm producing capacities
  c. both a and b above
  d. none of the above

___ 23. Age of menarche is influenced by
  a. nutrition
  b. exercise
  c. drug use
  d. radiation

___ 24. Adolescent males and females differ in which of the following physical characteristics?
  a. voice
  b. lean muscle mass
  c. structure of pelvic bones
  d. all of the above

___ 25. What rare but serious problem has been linked to the use of tampons?
  a. TSS
  b. AGS
  c. TFS
  d. ERT

PART V CLARIFYING YOUR VALUES

Puberty and adolescence are difficult periods developmentally for boys and girls. Try to recall the developmental changes that occurred during your adolescence. In the exercise that follows, identify how you felt about those changes which were occurring during that period of your life.

Legend

Timing — E = Early; A = Average; L = Late; NA = Not applicable

Gender — F = Female; M = Male; BS = Both sexes

Affect — EM = Embarrassed; SC = Self-conscious; CO = Comfortable;
SS = Self-satisfied; VA = Vain

Instructions

Place a checkmark (✓) in the appropriate spaces. If change is not applicable check NA and disregard the remainder of the line. Use comments to elaborate on feelings, etc.

Feelings about Developmental Changes

Developmental changes	Gender	Timing				Affect*					Comments
		NA	E	A	L	EM	SC	CO	SS	VA	
Growth spurt	BS										
Pubic hair	BS										
Axillary hair	BS										
Body hair	BS										
Sexual sensations	BS										
Erotic thoughts	BS										
Masturbation	BS										
Sexual activity with partner	BS										
Orgasm	BS										
Breast enlargement	F										
Rounding of hips and buttocks	F										
Widening of pelvis	F										
Menarche	F										
Vaginal secretions	F										
Vaginal lubrication	F										

*Feelings, attitudes, emotions about changes

Feelings about Developmental Changes (continued)

Developmental changes	Gender	Timing				Affect*					Comments
		NA	E	A	L	EM	SC	CO	SS	VA	
Voice deepening	M										
Penis and scrotum enlargement	M										
Transient breast swelling	M										
Increased muscle mass	M										
Widening of chest and shoulders	M										
Facial hair	M										
Chest hair	M										
Penile erections	M										
Wet dreams	M										
Others											

PART VI ANSWERS TO REVIEW QUIZ

1. True. See text p. 152.
2. True. See text p. 153.
3. False. See text p. 155.
4. False. See text p. 158.
5. True. See text p. 162.
6. True. See text p. 163.
7. True. See text p. 169.
8. False. See text p. 170.
9. False. See text p. 170.
10. True. See text p. 172.
11. (c) See text p. 152.
12. (d) See text p. 153.
13. (b) See text p. 153.
14. (d) See text p. 155.
15. (c) See text p. 155.
16. (a) See text p. 155.
17. (a) See text p. 156.
18. (b) See text p. 157.
19. (c) See text p. 158.
20. (b) See text p. 158.
21. (d) See text p. 159.
22. (c) See text p. 162.
23. (a) See text p. 164.
24. (d) See text pp. 167-169.
25. (a) See text p. 168.

PART TWO/PSYCHOSOCIAL PERSPECTIVES

7

Developmental Sexuality: A Psychosocial View

INTRODUCTION

This chapter examines the psychological and social factors that influence our sexual development at various stages in our lives. It focuses on three current theoretical viewpoints of gender development, and on the development of sexuality in childhood, adolescence, and adulthood. The chapter especially highlights Freud's theory of sexual development and the learning theorists' views related to sexual development.

PART I LEARNING OBJECTIVES

At the conclusion of this chapter, you should be able to:

1. Differentiate between gender identity and gender role.
2. Identify the three current theoretical viewpoints regarding gender development and describe each.
3. Describe the typical patterns of sexuality during the following developmental periods:
   a. Infancy (birth - end of first year)
   b. Early childhood (ages 2-5)
   c. School-age (ages 6-11)
   d. Adolescence (ages 12-19)
   e. Early adulthood (ages 20-29)
   f. Middle adulthood (ages 40-59)
   g. Late adulthood (ages 60+)
4. Explain Freud's theory of sexual development in terms of the five stages of psychosexual development.
5. Contrast the learning theory models of Classical Conditioning (Pavlov), Operant Conditioning (Thorndike, Watson and Skinner), and Social Learning (Bandura) with that of Freud's theory of psychosexual development.

PART II IMPORTANT TERMS AND NAMES TO KNOW

A. Fill in the missing word or words.

1. __________ __________ is the inner sense or conviction a person has of being male or female. (177) — gender identity

2. Behavior that conveys to others that an individual is either male or female is called __________ __________. (177) — gender role

3. The process in which parents and others react differently to boys and girls and reinforce different behaviors for the two sexes is known as __________ __________. (178) — differential socialization

4. __________ was a term used by Freud to label an instinct that strives for sensual pleasure (i.e., sexual desire). (179) — libido

5. The __________ __________ is the first year of life in which sexual energies are focused in the region of the mouth.* (179) — oral stage

6. The period when sensual pleasure is derived from eliminative functions is called the __________ __________.* (179) — anal stage

7. The period when a child's sexual energies are focused on the genitals is called the __________ __________.* (179) — phallic stage

8. The sexual attraction of a young boy to his mother is known as the __________ __________.* (179) — Oedipus complex

9. The unconscious fear in boys about the loss of their penises as a terrible form of punishment is called __________ __________.* (179) — castration anxiety

*According to Freudian theory

10. The sexual attraction of a young girl toward her father is called the __________ __________.* (179) — Electra complex

11. The period when sexual impulses are sublimated into nonsexual behaviors and interests is called the __________ __________.* (180) — latency stage

12. The last stage when the adolescent focuses sexual interest on heterosexual relations is called the __________ __________.* (180) — genital stage

B. Match the person(s) with the research or theory.

Researcher(s) and/or Theorist(s)	Research and/or Theory	Key
___ 1. Milton Diamond (178)	a. found differences in incidence of masturbation between teen males and females	Kinsey
___ 2. John Money (178)	b. classical conditioning	Pavlov
___ 3. Sigmund Freud (180)	c. learning influences gender development	Money
___ 4. Alfred Kinsey (193)	d. concept of sexual latency	Freud
___ 5. Robert Sorenson (196)	e. prenatal hormones organize sex differences in brain	Diamond
___ 6. Zelnick and Kantner (196)	f. operant conditioning	Skinner
___ 7. Jung and Erikson (198)	g. what is learned depends on prestige and power of other person	Bandura
___ 8. Gail Sheehy (198)	h. developmental aspects of adulthood	Jung and Erikson
___ 9. Ivan Pavlov (183)	i. teenage females' sexual behavior	Zelnick and Kantner
___ 10. B. F. Skinner (183)	j. teenage male and female sexual behavior	Sorenson
___ 11. Albert Bandura (184)	k. adult developmental stages as passage through predictable crises	Sheehy

*According to Freudian theory

PART III SELF-TESTING--A PROGRAMMED APPROACH

1. The theory that views gender development as being shaped by the personal models and the cultural influences to which the young child is exposed and rewarded is
   a. Learning Theory (Go to #2)
   b. Cognitive-Developmental Theory (Go to #3)
   c. Biosocial Interaction Theory (Go to #4)
   d. Psychoanalytical Theory (Go to #5)

2. Learning Theory suggests that a child learns to model the same-sex parent's behavior because imitation of that behavior is rewarded. You are correct. (Go to #6)

3. Cognitive-Developmental Theory considers gender development as a parallel to cognitive or intellectual development. As cognition of gender unfolds, gender identity is developed. The gender-appropriate behavior is learned by observation and imitation of others but not for rewards, rather to maintain both gender identity and gender roles. You are incorrect. (Go to #2)

4. Biosocial Interaction proponents view the process of gender development as an interaction between the biological and psychosocial factors in which prenatal programming influences subsequent patterns during childhood and adolescence. It does not include the operant conditioning component of learning theory (i.e., reward of appropriate behavior). You are incorrect. (Go to #2)

5. Psychoanalytical Theory is based on Freud's belief that sexual feelings develop from a predictable series of stages. It does not focus on external factors such as models and is not based on learning theory. You are incorrect. (Go to #2)

6. Which of the following explanations of infantile genital play does existing evidence tend to support?
   a. The behavior is nothing more than a simple exploration of body parts with an equal likelihood that equally accessible parts will be touched as frequently as other parts. (Go to #7)
   b. There is a sexual component with a genuine sense of pleasure resulting from such behavior; this leads to repeated self-stimulation. (Go to #8)
   c. There is an innate need to reduce sexual tension; touching returns the infant to the homeostatic state. (Go to #9)
   d. Genital play is mainly the infant's sensory response to genito-urinary tension caused by pressure of a full bladder or wet diaper irritation. (Go to #10)

7. Simple exploration of body parts as an explanation does not hold up when investigators observe the response of infants to their genitals being stimulated versus stimulation of other body parts (i.e., babies express joy when genitals are touched). You are incorrect. (Go to #8)

8. Investigators have observed that babies express joy, smile, and coo when their genitals are stimulated and show extreme annoyance when their efforts to touch their own genitals are interrupted. You are correct. (Go to #11)

9. Homeostasis is not a well accepted notion concerning genital self-stimulation. It is more commonly used to explain responses necessary to maintain or restore biochemical balance in the body. You are incorrect. (Go to #8)

10. Babies have been observed fondling their genitals following bladder evacuation and after wet diapers have been removed. This self-stimulation of the genitals is not limited to periods of bladder pressure or urethral irritation. You are incorrect. (Go to #8)

11. Sexual experimentation among children of the same sex or of the opposite sex is common. Which of the following descriptions helps to explain the behavior?
    a. It is a normal rebellious reaction to parental warnings about engaging in "bad" behavior (i.e., testing the forbidden). (Go to #12)
    b. Children are seeking information about how similar and/or different they are from others. (Go to #13)
    c. It is a necessary and valuable developmental experience. (Go to #14)
    d. All of the above are good explanations. (Go to #15)

12. Wanting to see what they can get away with is one of the purposes of this behavior but not necessarily the only one or the most important. Therefore, your answer is correct but not the best one. (Go to #15)

13. Knowledge seeking is purposeful; however, it is one of the purposes served by this behavior and not necessarily the only one or the most important one. Therefore, your answer is correct but not the best one. (Go to #15)

14. Most experts agree that childhood sex play is probably a valuable psychosocial experience in developmental terms; however, it is too limited an explanation to stand on its own. Therefore, your answer is correct but not the best one. (Go to #15)

15. All of the purposes described above help to explain the behavior; however, none, on its own, is complete enough. The first two are inextricably interrelated since taboos are more enticing to a child than sanctioned practices (i.e., forbidden knowledge is more alluring than easily available knowledge). Most experts feel that sexual experimentation is not psychologically harmful but is probably a valuable experience. You are correct because your answer is the most complete one of the group. (Go to #16)

16. In adolescence, sexual decision-making often results in conflicts between
    a. cultural norms and personal values as factors that are reflected in the decision-making process (Go to #17)
    b. moral reasoning and romantic attachment (Go to #18)
    c. psychological readiness and fear of negative consequences (Go to #19)
    d. need for individual freedom and need to be like friends (Go to #20)

17. Cultural norms and personal values are factors reflected in the decision-making process. They are not necessarily in conflict. You are incorrect. (Go to #20)

18. Moral reasoning and romantic attachments are factors that are involved in the process of deciding about sexual options. They are not necessarily in conflict with one another. You are incorrect. (Go to #20)

19. Psychological readiness and fear of negative consequences are factors that affect teenagers' sexual decision-making but are not necessarily in conflict with one another. You are incorrect. (Go to #20)

20. The adolescent's need for freedom is usually accompanied by a need to be like his or her friends. These two needs are very often in conflict. You are correct.

PART IV REVIEW QUIZ

A. True or False

___ 1. The purely psychological state experienced privately in a person's feelings and self-awareness of being male or female is known as gender role.

___ 2. The biosocial viewpoint of gender development stresses the existence of certain critical periods in the overall process of sexual development.

___ 3. There is little reliable data about sexual behavior during childhood.

___ 4. The negative messages that children get from their parents when they touch their genitals are considered by many authorities to be among the earliest causes of sexual problems in later years.

___ 5. Freud's concept of a period of sexual latency during late childhood is one of the longest standing accepted theories.

___ 6. Sexual fantasy, especially during adolescence, is mentally unhealthy because it distorts the real world for the adolescent and erodes coping skills in later life.

___ 7. There is a trend toward a higher incidence of masturbation among young women since Kinsey's studies during the 1950s.

___ 8. There is a definite trend recently toward marriage at an earlier age than in the past two decades.

___ 9. Most young adults today believe that virginity is the preferred sexual state before selecting a marriage partner.

___ 10. Despite cultural myths, the need for sexual activity and all that it brings to the individual does not disappear in old age.

B. Multiple Choice--Select the Best Answer

___ 11. The outward expression of one's maleness or femaleness is
a. gender identity
b. gender role
c. gender preference
d. gender orientation

___ 12. The treatment of boys and girls differently from the moment of birth is believed to influence
a. gender identity
b. gender role
c. differential socialization
d. both a and b above

___ 13. John Money and his co-workers, who investigated gender development, studied which of the following types of subjects?
a. a clustered random sample of teenagers
b. randomly selected siblings
c. randomly selected, institutionalized transvestites
d. matched pairs of pseudohermaphrodites

___ 14. Ultrasound studies of male fetuses have shown
a. reflex erections occur before birth
b. oral gratification in utero
c. both a and b above
d. none of the above

___ 15. Parent-child bonding includes
a. nursing
b. bathing
c. dressing
d. all of the above

___ 16. Children become aware of parental attitudes toward genital play as early as
a. 1 year old
b. 3 years old
c. 6 years old
d. 10 years old

___ 17. Children in our society usually begin asking questions about how babies are made and how birth occurs by the time they are
a. 2 years old
b. 3 years old
c. 4 years old
d. 5 years old

___ 18. Most children have a basic understanding of anatomic differences between the sexes and show a strong sense of modesty about nudity by the time they
a. go to school
b. play with other children
c. view their parents nude
d. begin to talk

___ 19. Psychological harm can come to children who participate in sex play and who
a. enjoy playing with their siblings
b. enjoy playing with members of the same sex
c. receive harsh parental reaction
d. all of the above

___ 20. Parents often react with more of a double-standard (sexually) to the sexual activity of their children when they
a. start school
b. enter puberty
c. begin dating
d. go away to college

___ 21. Sexual fantasies and dreams in adolescence are often
a. a way of adding pleasure to sexual activity
b. a substitute for the real thing
c. an accompaniment to masturbation
d. all of the above

___ 22. Teenagers who worry about being homosexual may deal with it by
a. avoiding same sex contacts and going out only with members of the opposite sex
b. withdrawing from all sexual situations
c. viewing themselves as bisexual
d. all of the above

___ 23. According to Erikson, a central task for the young adult is to
a. accept earlier homosexual behaviors
b. date as many people of the opposite sex as possible
c. develop the capacity for intimacy
d. all of the above

___ 24. Which of the following common patterns of sexual behavior involves judging the sexual experience on the basis of frequency, variety, and performance proficiency?
a. the experimenter
b. the seeker
c. the user
d. the traditionalist

___ 25. The sense that "time is running out" and the need to reappraise one's goals, accomplishments, and experiences often results in a phenomenon called
a. passages
b. mid-life crisis
c. tour de force
d. career reevaluation

PART V CLARIFYING YOUR VALUES

Psychological and social factors influence our sexual development at various stages of our lives. Some seem more significant than others. Many of these influences can stereotype our ideas about what constitutes maleness and femaleness.

The exercise that follows is intended to give you an opportunity to reflect upon your own psychosocial sexual development. In doing so, you may be able to clarify the values you presently hold regarding maleness and femaleness. Place a check (√) in the appropriate boxes to indicate your recollection of the developmental stage in which each of the knowledge, attitudes, and/or behavior manifested itself, the social influences that intervened, and your current feelings regarding that episode in your life.

Legend

Developmental Stage	Social Influences	Feelings
IN = Infancy	PA = Parent(s)	+ Positive
EC = Early childhood	PE = Peers	= Neutral
SA = School age	SI = Siblings	- Negative
TA = Teenage	TE = Teachers	
AD = Adulthood	CL = Clergy/Church/Religion	

Recollections about Psychosocial Sexual Development

Knowledge/Attitudes/Behavior	Developmental Stage					Social Influences					Feelings		
	IN	EC	SA	TA	AD	PA	PE	SI	TE	CL	+	=	-
Gender identity													
Gender role													
Bonding													
Genital self-stimulation													
Sexual play with others													
Understanding of anatomical differences													
How birth occurs													
Masturbation to orgasm													
Homosexual contacts													
Erection or vaginal lubrication													
Sexual fantasy													
Petting													
Attempts at coitus													
Successful coitus													
"Falling in love"													
Independence from parents													

Now that you've completed the exercise, respond to the following questions.

1. As a parent, how would you handle situations with your children which you can recall having a negative feeling about now?

2. What sexual values would you want your daughter to grow up with?

3. What sexual values would you want your son to grow up with?

4. Are there any differences between questions 2 and 3? If so, why? If not, why not?

PART VI ANSWERS TO REVIEW QUIZ

1. False. See text p. 177.
2. True. See text p. 178.
3. True. See text p. 182.
4. True. See text pp. 186, 189.
5. False. See text p. 190.
6. False. See text p. 191.
7. True. See text p. 193.
8. False. See text p. 198.
9. False. See text p. 198.
10. True. See text pp. 201-202.
11. (b) See text p. 177.
12. (d) See text pp. 181-182.
13. (d) See text pp. 178-182.
14. (a) See text p. 182.
15. (d) See text pp. 182-185.
16. (b) See text pp. 186-187.
17. (c) See text p. 187.
18. (a) See text p. 188.
19. (c) See text p. 189.
20. (b) See text p. 192.
21. (d) See text p. 191.
22. (d) See text p. 197.
23. (c) See text p. 198.
24. (a) See text p. 199.
25. (b) See text p. 200.

8
Gender Roles

INTRODUCTION

This chapter reviews the trends that have affected gender roles and examines old attitudes toward sex differences, child rearing practices, notions about masculinity and femininity, and society's view of gender role behavior. The chapter explores these issues as they influence the experience of being male or female.

PART I LEARNING OBJECTIVES

At the conclusion of this chapter, you should be able to:

1. List the traits that are most often used to characterize the typical man and woman in our culture and discuss the potential harm these stereotypes can cause.
2. Identify the major patterns of gender role socialization at each developmental level.
3. Define androgyny and describe the reasons that there is no firm agreement among researchers about what constitutes an androgynous person.
4. Discuss the determination of psychological differences that exist between the sexes and explain the use of an alternative ("brain-based") approach to investigate differences between the sexes.
5. Describe how gender role expectations in adult life affect marriage, work, politics, and play.
6. List the biological and psychological factors that have been suggested as causes of transsexualism.
7. Contrast the gender role expectations between American and Mangaian cultures and analyze their impact upon sexual attitudes, behavior, and stereotypes.
8. Describe the double standard as it applies to sexual behavior in our society.
9. Predict some of the expectations for gender role in the future American culture twenty years from now.
10. Describe some of the ways that parents can initiate nonsexist child-rearing practices with their own children.

PART II IMPORTANT TERMS AND NAMES TO KNOW

Fill in the missing word, words, or names.

1.	Fixed, conventional beliefs based on over-simplified evidence or uncritical judgments are known as __________. (206)	stereotypes
2.	__________ is the combined presence of stereotyped feminine and masculine characteristics in one person. (216)	androgyny
3.	A(n) __________ is an individual who feels incongruity between anatomical sex and gender identity. (218)	transsexual
4.	A(n) __________ is an individual who receives sexual gratification and release from anxiety by dressing in the clothing of the opposite sex. (219)	transvestite
5.	Researchers __________ and __________ studied androgyny and found androgynous individuals display more self-esteem, achievement orientation, and social competence than people who are nonandrogynous. (216)	Spence/Helmreich
6.	Researchers __________ and __________ reviewed books and articles on sex differences in children and described the status of the research on psychological differences between the sexes. (217)	Maccoby/Jacklin
7.	__________ __________ was the first American to achieve notoriety for undergoing sex change surgery. (218)	Christine Jorgensen
8.	__________ __________ published a book that gives very straightforward advice to parents on how to decrease the effects of gender role stereotypes by nonsexist child-rearing practices. (209)	Letty Pogrebin

PART III SELF-TESTING--A PROGRAMMED APPROACH

1. During the last 25 years there has been considerable scientific interest in studying differences and similarities between the sexes. The motivation for this interest stems from
   a. the Women's Movement which has increased the awareness about sex discrimination and sexism (Go to #2)
   b. recent trends which have challenged former distinctions between the sexes (Go to #3)
   c. so many varied beliefs about sex differences which have influenced society (Go to #4)
   d. all of the above (Go to #5)

2. The Women's Movement has raised the consciousness of both men and women to the need for sexual equality. However, it is but one of the motivations during the past 25 years for increased scientific interest in sex differences. You are only partially correct. (Go to #5)

3. More women work outside the home than 25 years ago; unisex hairstyles, clothing, jewelry, etc. are more fashionable today; anatomic structures is no longer fixed (e.g., transsexual surgery), etc. These are some of the recent trends which have altered the traditional distinctions between the sexes; however, these trends are only part of the motivation for scientific interest in sex differences. You are incorrect. (Go to #5)

4. Various beliefs about sex differences in traits, talents, abilities, temperaments, and skills have greatly influenced social, political, and economic systems throughout history. However, these beliefs and the emerging challenges they pose have been only part of the motivation to pursue scientific inquiry into sex differences and similarities. You are incorrect. (Go to #5)

5. All of these have had an impact on the increased interest in the scientific community about differences and similarities between the sexes. There are a number of reasons for this increase. You are correct. (Go to #6)

6. Tradition has held that it is highly desirable for men and women to behave in ways that match the expectations of their culture. The traditional approach to studying masculinity and femininity viewed these traits as opposites. As a result, most psychological tests were designed to measure masculinity and femininity
   a. as a single masculinity-femininity scale (Go to #7)
   b. as a personality profile (Go to #8)
   c. as a sexual orientation inventory (Go to #9)
   d. as a life-style analysis (Go to #10)

7. Since it was assumed that if you possess "feminine" characteristics you can't have "masculine" ones and vice versa, a single scale for masculinity and femininity was used. It was assumed that if you scored high on certain traits judged as masculine, you also had a general lack of femininity. You are correct. (Go to #11)

8. Personality profiles do not provide clues to gender roles. The degree of masculinity-femininity tells little if anything about personality. You are incorrect. (Go to #7)

9. Sexual orientation is an indication of an individual's preference for sexual partners and does not apply to gender role. You are incorrect. (Go to #7)

10. Life-style analysis is a technique used to determine ways in which people deal or cope with the tasks of living. Life-styles are not measures of gender role although some life-styles are associated with masculine-feminine characteristics in our culture. You are incorrect. (Go to #7)

11. During early infancy, male babies receive
    a. more verbal contact with their mothers than female babies (Go to #12)
    b. more physical contact with their mothers than female babies (Go to #13)
    c. more visual contact with their mothers than female babies (Go to #14)
    d. more quick attention to their cries than female babies (Go to #15)

12. Mothers talk more to their female infants than to their male infants. You are incorrect. (Go to #13)

13. Mothers touch, pick up, hold, and play more with their male infants than with their female infants. This may account for the increased physical activity among males. You are correct. (Go to #16)

14. Mothers look more at their female infants than at their male infants. You are incorrect. (Go to #13)

15. Mothers and fathers respond differently to the cries of their baby girls than to their baby boys. Perhaps it's considered a way to "toughen up" the male and program him for greater independence since parents react more quickly to the cries of their baby girls. This may unintentionally program the girls for greater dependency and passivity. You are incorrect. (Go to #13)

16. Androgyny seems to have some distinct <u>disadvantages</u> as well as potential advantages. The disadvantages include
    a. lower self-esteem (Go to #17)
    b. lower achievement orientation (Go to #18)
    c. higher level of emotional problems (Go to #19)
    d. lower problem-solving skills (Go to #20)

17. Androgynous individuals seem to display more self-esteem than people who are strong in either masculinity or femininity. You are incorrect. (Go to #19)

18. Androgynous men and women are more achievement oriented than their non-androgynous cohorts. You are incorrect. (Go to #19)

19. One of the disadvantages androgyny holds for its adherents is the fact that androgynous people have more problem-drinking behavior, are less in control of their behavior, and are more apt to seek out psychotherapy. They do appear to have a higher level of emotional problems than masculine males and feminine females. You are correct.

20. Androgyny does not appear to make a difference in behavioral effectiveness or problem-solving abilities. Androgynous people have neither better nor worse problem-solving skills than masculine males or feminine females. You are incorrect. (Go to #19)

PART IV REVIEW QUIZ

A. True or False

___ 1. Most behavioral scientists view masculinity and femininity as separate characteristics that coexist to some degree in every individual.

___ 2. The process of gender role socialization begins even before a baby is born.

___ 3. Many of the learning materials used by children in school foster gender role stereotypes.

___ 4. When a teenage boy shows "feminine" interests or traits, he is often considered to be a potential homosexual.

___ 5. Many females are led to believe that achievement detracts from their popularity.

___ 6. Studies suggest that about half of all college students are androgynous.

___ 7. Males are conditioned to equate their masculinity with their sexual experience.

___ 8. Sexual behavior has been strongly influenced by gender role stereotypes.

___ 9. Psychotherapy has been generally successful in resolving the transsexual's basic distress about being trapped in the wrong body.

___ 10. Studies in the psychology of sex differences show that males and females are more different than alike psychologically.

B. Multiple Choice--Select the Best Answer

___ 11. Sexual stereotypes can be harmful because they
   a. can alter gender identity in boys and girls, causing anxiety
   b. lead to gender role confusion in boys and girls
   c. lead to erroneous judgments and generalizations and thus affect how people treat one another
   d. create emotional problems requiring professional intervention

___ 12. Masculinity and femininity are defined as
 a. the sexual attraction one has to members of the opposite sex
 b. the degree to which a person matches cultural expectations of how males and females should behave or look
 c. traits measured by standardized psychological tests that compare one person's responses to those of large groups of men and women
 d. because many sexual stereotypes are based on assumptions about the nature of masculinity and femininity, it is difficult to define these two terms

___ 13. Parents of newborn infants describe sons as
 a. less attentive than daughters
 b. less active than daughters
 c. more dependent than daughters
 d. stronger and larger than daughters

___ 14. Core gender identity is well established by the time a child reaches
 a. the end of the first year of life
 b. the age of 3 years old
 c. school age
 d. puberty

___ 15. Gender role socialization is affected by
 a. toys for children
 b. picture books for children
 c. television
 d. all of the above

___ 16. Gender role stereotypes are fostered in school classrooms by
 a. the use of elementary school readers that show male figures more frequently than females
 b. history lessons that portray a male-dominated world
 c. assigning boys and girls different chores based on presumptions about gender roles
 d. all of the above

___ 17. Although girls show better school performance in all subjects until the adolescent years, their performance after puberty declines due in large part to the impression that
 a. academic achievement may reduce or lessen their femininity
 b. men are less likely to marry women who are intelligent
 c. popular girls are not the intelligent ones
 d. all of the above

___ 18. Gender role stereotypes usually come into full impact during a person's
 a. childhood
 b. adolescence
 c. adulthood
 d. old age

___ 19. In general, married men tend to be physically and mentally healthier than their wives because
a. they have two sources of gratification--work and family; their wives usually have only one
b. their wives find raising children and doing housework emotionally fulfilling but physically exhausting
c. the role of housewife brings their wives into contact with more mental and physical illness stressors
d. working wives do not encourage their husbands to share equally in the housework and care of the children and are therefore under greater physical and mental strain

___ 20. Most people are not 100 percent masculine or feminine since they demonstrate traits that are socially labelled as belonging to the opposite sex. When someone exhibits a combination of stereotypical traits, we refer to that person as
a. androgynous
b. a transsexual
c. a homosexual
d. a transvestite

___ 21. Boys excel over girls in
a. analytical ability
b. doing repetitive tasks
c. mathematical ability
d. self-esteem

___ 22. Girls excel over boys in
a. verbal abilities
b. social abilities
c. resistance to social pressure to conform
d. response to aspects of their environment that require vision

___ 23. Transsexual surgery is
a. usually preceded by a trial period of one to two years
b. usually preceded by hormone therapy
c. usually preceded by periodic evaluation by a psychiatrist or psychologist
d. all of the above

___ 24. Many men and women are beginning to realize that achieving the pleasure that they both want from sex requires
a. a reevaluation of the double standard
b. knowledge of the sexual response cycle
c. realizing that sex is not something one person does to another but something done together as equal participants
d. giving up gender role stereotypes in favor of androgynous life-styles

___ 25. Cross-cultural evidence indicates that many male-female differences found in our society are derived from
a. biological predispositions
b. psychosexual development
c. social and economic conditions
d. stereotypic expectations

PART V CLARIFYING YOUR VALUES

The exercise that follows will give you an opportunity to express your feelings and beliefs about gender roles in our society. Although the activity will give you only a rough measure of what you believe about male-female roles, it should help to clarify your values about gender roles. The column on the left is a list of traits and activities that have been associated with gender roles. In the right-hand column, you are to check the gender assignment you would personally assign to each of the items in the left-hand column. Be honest; what you really feel is more important than what you think you _should_ feel.

Trait/Activity	Gender Assignment		
	Male	Female	Androgynous
Aggressive			
Sensitive			
Competitive			
Nurturing			
Verbal			
Logical			
Robust			
Fragile			
Gentle			
Rough			
Passive			
Sexy			
Artist			
Athlete			
Dancer			
Boss			
Nurse			
Teacher			
Leader			
Physician			
Mechanic			
Breadwinner			
Homemaker			

What person, persons, groups, institutions, etc. influenced your beliefs?

Review this exercise. Think about your responses. Complete the following sentences:

I learned that I . . .

I was surprised that I . . .

PART VI ANSWERS TO REVIEW QUIZ

1. True. See text p. 207.
2. True. See text p. 207.
3. True. See text p. 212.
4. True. See text p. 211.
5. True. See text p. 213.
6. False. See text p. 216.
7. True. See text p. 221.
8. True. See text p. 221.
9. False. See text p. 219.
10. False. See text p. 217.
11. (c) See text p. 206.
12. (d) See text p. 206.
13. (d) See text p. 208.
14. (b) See text p. 208.
15. (d) See text pp. 208-211.
16. (d) See text p. 212.
17. (d) See text p. 213.
18. (c) See text p. 214.
19. (a) See text p. 215.
20. (a) See text p. 216.
21. (c) See text p. 217.
22. (a) See text pp. 217-218.
23. (d) See text pp. 219-220.
24. (c) See text pp. 222-223.
25. (d) See text p. 221.

9
Loving and Being Loved

INTRODUCTION

The topic of love, until fairly recently, has been discussed by poets, writers, and philosophers. Few scientists or academicians have dealt with the subject in any detail. This chapter focuses on the complicated relationships between love, sex, and marriage.

PART I LEARNING OBJECTIVES

At the conclusion of this chapter, you should be able to:

1. Define love and distinguish it from sexual desire.
2. Describe what happens to love relationships when respect and caring are missing elements in them.
3. Distinguish between love as a healthy relationship with growth potential and love as a form of dependency or addiction.
4. Discuss the psychological theories about the nature of romantic love and outline a conceptual model of the Romantic Love Cycle.
5. Identify the six primary types of romantic love, according to Lee.
6. Explain the basis of companionate love.
7. State the two types of evidence that support the view that there is a biological component of love.
8. Define intimacy and contrast relational sex with impersonal sex.
9. Identify the sources of potential conflict among personal values involved in sexual decision-making.
10. Discuss the relationship of love and marriage and explain the mate selection process in our culture.

PART II IMPORTANT TERMS AND NAMES TO KNOW

Fill in the missing word, words, or names.

1. The Art of Loving, written by __________ __________, was a classic book that has exerted a major influence on contemporary ideas about love. (226) — Erich Fromm

2. The view that some love relationships are dependency relationships and therefore a form of addiction was promulgated by __________ and __________. (226-227) — Peele/Brodsky

3. __________ is a word coined by __________ __________ to describe a blind, intense kind of love outside the person's rational control. (229) — limerence Dorothy Tennov

4. A sociologist who developed the categorization of the six primary types of romantic love was __________ __________. (230) — Alan Lee

5. __________ is a type of love that is based on physical attraction. (230) — eros

6. __________ is a type of love that is a playful, casual variety without high levels of commitment. (230) — ludus

7. __________ is a type of love that has no identifiable starting point but emerges slowly as warmth and affection. (230) — storge

8. __________ is a stormy love that is characterized by turbulent highs and lows. (230) — mania

9. __________ is a practical type of love. (230) — pragma

10. __________ is an undemanding, patient, kind of spiritual love. (230) — agape

11. A soothing, secure, reality-based love usually characteristic of marriage and long-term relationships is known as __________ __________. (235) — companionate love

12. Psychologist __________ __________ devised a theory based on the fact that emotions are accompanied by physiological responses and we distinguish among them by how we interpret or label what we are experiencing. (236) — Stanley Schacter

PART III SELF-TESTING--A PROGRAMMED APPROACH

1. In any type of love, the one element that is essential is
   a. passion for the person (Go to #2)
   b. friendship of the person (Go to #3)
   c. caring about the person (Go to #4)
   d. dependency on the person (Go to #5)

2. Passion is a very narrowly focused form of desire. It often is based on the need to fulfill one's own needs by using someone else. Love is not so single-minded. You are incorrect. (Go to #4)

3. Friendship is a steadier basis for love since it is based on trust; however, it is too narrowly focused. Love can emerge from friendship but is not the essential element in love. You are incorrect. (Go to #4)

4. Unless genuine caring for the person is present, what appears to be love may be just sexual desire or infatuation. In sexual desire, the caring is minimal, perhaps peripheral or an afterthought, but not a central part of the feeling. You are correct. (Go to #6)

5. Dependency is what happens when caring is missing from a love relationship. Dependency is a means to fill a void, it is self-centered and not designed to preserve the integrity of the loved person. You are incorrect. (Go to #4)

6. Limerence is a term coined to describe a particularly powerful form of romantic love. It is characterized by
   a. a preoccupation with thoughts of the loved one and the belief that only this person can satisfy the lover's needs (Go to #7)
   b. being possessive or overly jealous of the other's growth and expansion of interests (Go to #8)
   c. its immediacy and its propensity to be ignited or extinguished quickly (Go to #9)
   d. its slow and gradual emergence from a friendship relationship (Go to #10)

7. Limerence is completely outside of rational control so that the limerent lover dotes on every word or gesture in hope of approval and in fear of rejection. It is an affliction of being "love-struck," or being preoccupied with the other person. You are correct. (Go to #11)

8. Possessiveness and jealousy may be part of the limerent lover's mood at times; however, it depends almost totally on the actions of the loved one. If the actions do not precipitate this type of response, it may very well be uncharacteristic of limerence. You are incorrect. (Go to #7)

9. Most forms of romantic love have some form of time sequence associated with them. The form that is based primarily on physical sexual intensity is most likely to quickly ignite and just as quickly fizzle out. Limerence does not necessarily focus on sexual magnetism, but on psychological need gratification. You are incorrect. (Go to #7)

10. Slow and gradual development of romantic love from friendship is a very stable and solid type of love that can withstand crises. Limerence has little of this stable quality as it fluctuates with the mood of the lover which, in turn, depends on the behavior of the loved one. You are incorrect. (Go to #7)

11. The pivotal time in the phases of the Romantic Love Cycle is characterized by lovers beginning to notice imperfections in each other. This generally occurs during the
    a. Love Readiness Phase (Go to #12)
    b. Falling in Love Phase (Go to #13)
    c. Being in Love Phase (Go to #14)
    d. Transitional Love Phase (Go to #15)

12. Love readiness is a preliminary state in which an individual's mind views love as rewarding, is longing for interpersonal intimacy, and is experiencing an element of sexual frustration. They are more likely to make concessions during this phase and be less conscious of imperfections in a potential loved one. You are incorrect. (Go to #15)

13. Falling in love is a process which starts in many ways including dating, physical closeness, and friendships. The excitement of getting to know someone intimately during this phase usually obliterates the person's failings while exaggerating the real or hoped for virtues. It is unlikely that lovers will begin to notice imperfections while falling in love. You are incorrect. (Go to #15)

14. Being in love usually finds the romantic lover sexually attracted to the loved one and possibly caught in the grips of limerence. Given the intensity of this experience, it is highly unlikely that imperfections will be noticed. You are incorrect. (Go to #15)

15. The transitional phase is the time when the initial excitement of knowing someone and the heat of passion begin to lessen. Lovers begin to notice imperfections that were previously overlooked. Lovers begin to test one another and power struggles often ensue. It is indeed a pivotal time. You are correct. (Go to #16)

16. Love and marriage are not synonymous but they are linked in several important ways. Which of the following statements most accurately expresses the cultural value inherent in the relationship between love and marriage in our American culture?
    a. Couples who live together without the benefit of marriage are more committed to each other than married couples because they trust the relationship without the security that legal marriage brings to it. (Go to #17)
    b. Arranged marriages are initially void of love because they are manipulated by persons external to the relationship. Devotion and responsibility grow as the marriage develops. Love is not essential to its (marriage) success. (Go to #18)
    c. Love before marriage is the cultural value that sets the stage for mate selection as <u>sine qua non</u>. (Go to #19)
    d. Love is so irrational that we need to develop a scientific analysis for the selection of a mate such as the computer dating services. Love can occur within marriage when we are happiest in equitable relationships. Therefore, we're better off marrying by intelligent analysis rather than emotional choices. (Go to #20)

17. Some couples who live together without the benefit of marriage are more loving (i.e., caring) than couples who are married. But "cohabitation" is no more a guarantee of respect and caring than a marriage certificate is a guarantee that two people will successfully meet each other's needs. They are not mutually exclusive. You are incorrect. (Go to #19)

18. Arranged marriages are not part of our cultural pattern, even when ethnic and national origins are in their first American generation. In India, China, Japan, and parts of Africa and the Arab world, arranged marriages are common. You are incorrect. (Go to #19)

19. Our culture is unique in the emphasis it places on love before marriage. We are expected to select our mate for the rest of our lives largely on the basis of love. You are correct.

20. We are still too romantically committed to our sense of natural passion and the desire to be "one with our loved one," however irrational it may seem, to adopt a computer analysis of likely marriage candidates. Cognitively we "know" that it's riskier to marry someone with a markedly different background but it ends there. Most marriages are based on romantic love, not on statistics. You are incorrect. (Go to #19)

PART IV REVIEW QUIZ

<u>A. True or False</u>

___ 1. Caring and respect for the other person are central features of sexual passion.

___ 2. In romantic love, we tend to immerse ourselves almost completely in another person.

___ 3. Unlike other forms of romantic love, limerence is almost completely within our rational control.

___ 4. It is rare for a romantic love relationship to last for more than a few years.

___ 5. A biological basis for love can be demonstrated by the fact that genetically unrelated persons were drawn together to produce a diversified gene pool contributing to the survival of the species.

___ 6. Intimacy is similar to love in that the happiness of the other person is its principal concern.

___ 7. There is scientific evidence that establishes that sex is usually better if you're in love.

___ 8. There are forms of romantic love and companionate love in which there is no sexual contact.

___ 9. Men and women tend to be happiest in equitable relationships.

___ 10. Marital dissatisfaction tends to decrease the longer people stay married.

B. Multiple Choice--Select the Best Answer

___ 11. The central feature of love that is lacking in sexual desire is
a. passion
b. control
c. respect
d. self-fulfillment

___ 12. Fromm believed that people can only achieve a meaningful type of love if they have first reached a state of
a. self-realization
b. self-esteem
c. self-actualization
d. self-direction

___ 13. A basic characteristic of romantic love is the
a. intensity of passion for the other person
b. intensity of jealousy about the other person
c. distortion of time spent with the other person
d. distortion of objectivity about the other person

___ 14. When someone is labelled a "limerent lover" it usually suggests that the person is
a. head-over-heels in love with the other person
b. emotionally committed to the other person
c. spiritually attached to the other person
d. sexually obsessed with the other person

___ 15. Alan Lee assigned Greek and Latin names to six primary types of romantic love. The one that is more of an ideal than a reality is
a. ludus
b. storge
c. agape
d. eros

___ 16. In the Romantic Love-Cycle, the Love Readiness stage is characterized by which of the following elements?
a. Love is seen as rewarding
b. There is a longing for intimacy
c. There is a degree of sexual frustration
d. All of the above

___ 17. A common pathway to the Falling in Love stage is
a. love at first sight
b. being physically near a person
c. reading about someone's qualities
d. being told about someone's qualities

___ 18. The romantic lover at the Being in Love stage
a. may resort to masturbation to diffuse sexual impulses
b. may resort to strenuous physical exercise to diffuse sexual impulses
c. may be caught in the grips of limerence
d. all of the above

___ 19. Which of the following Romantic Love Cycle stages is pivotal because it is the time when lovers begin to notice imperfections in each other?
a. Being Out of Love
b. Falling Out of Love
c. Love in Transition
d. all of the above

___ 20. Companionate love is
a. the love shared by old people
b. sexless love
c. less turbulent and more predictable love than romantic love
d. all of the above

___ 21. Intimacy differs from love in that
a. the happiness of the other person is not the principal concern of intimacy
b. intimacy requires sexual contact
c. there are no boundaries for closeness or mutually agreeable set of expectations among intimate partners
d. you can be in love and not be intimate, but you can't be intimate and not be in love

___ 22. Under what conditions or circumstances can a love relationship exist without sexual interaction?
a. geographic separation
b. illness
c. conscious decision to abstain
d. all of the above

___ 23. Research on "equity theory" has shown that men and women generally marry someone
   a. with different physical attractiveness and similar intelligence
   b. with similar physical attractiveness and different intelligence
   c. with similar physical attractiveness and similar intelligence
   d. with different physical attractiveness and different intelligence

___ 24. Researchers have found that marital dissatisfaction tends to increase
   a. due to responsibilities of parenting
   b. the longer people have been married
   c. when women are employed outside of the home
   d. when romantic love shifts to companionate love

___ 25. It's generally accepted that in order to maintain love or help it grow, marriage partners must work at
   a. improving communication
   b. giving physical warmth
   c. sharing interests and responsibilities
   d. all of the above

PART V CLARIFYING YOUR VALUES

Each person approaches sexual decision making from a framework of personal values, beliefs, and experiences. We all start off with a particular set of values that have been influenced by our socialization and must, at one time or another, deal with conflicts that exist between our personal needs and those endorsed by our culture. Even more important are the built-in conflicts between the various personal needs we each have.

The exercise that follows is intended to help you judge the relative importance of your personal values in the hope that your sexual decisions may be more of a result of considered action rather than just letting the "decision" happen.

Rate the relative importance of the conflicting values presented on the continua on the following page. Place a check (√) along each continuum.

Value Conflicts

1	5	10
commitment		freedom

1	5	10
intimacy		privacy

1	5	10
permanence		sexual novelty

1	5	10
sexual fidelity		independence

What effect(s) will these personal values have upon your sexual decisions? The next part of this exercise may help clarify this issue.

In the table which follows, place a check in the column that represents the impact your value will have on your decision.

Effect of Values on Decisions

Decisions	Effect			Comments
	Major	Uncertain	Minimal	
Other person's happiness				
Own state of self-realization				
Sex without love				
Love without sex				
Impersonal or casual sex				
Relational or intimate sex				
Premarital sex				
Extramarital sex				
Living together				
Marriage				
Companionate love				
Others?				

PART VI ANSWERS TO REVIEW QUIZ

1. False. See text p. 226.
2. True. See text p. 228.
3. False. See text p. 229.
4. True. See text p. 235.
5. True. See text p. 236.
6. False. See text p. 236.
7. False. See text pp. 237-238.
8. True. See text p. 235.
9. True. See text p. 239.
10. False. See text p. 241.
11. (c) See text p. 226.
12. (a) See text p. 226.
13. (d) See text p. 228.
14. (a) See text p. 229.
15. (c) See text p. 230.
16. (d) See text pp. 231-232.
17. (b) See text p. 232.
18. (d) See text pp. 232-234
19. (c) See text p. 234.
20. (c) See text p. 235.
21. (a) See text p. 236.
22. (d) See text pp. 237-238.
23. (c) See text p. 239.
24. (b) See text p. 241.
25. (d) See text p. 241.

10
Sexual Fantasy

INTRODUCTION

Most people use fantasy to escape from the limits of their everyday lives. Through it, the real world is transformed in whatever way the fantasizer wishes. This chapter explores the functions of sexual fantasies and provides a classification for describing the most common types of fantasy patterns used by people to find adventure, excitement, and pleasure through individual mental excursions.

PART I LEARNING OBJECTIVES

At the conclusion of this chapter, you should be able to:

1. Define sexual fantasy and distinguish it from sexual desire.
2. State the most common forms of fantasies.
3. Identify the situations in which preferential fantasies can become troublesome.
4. List the most common functions of sexual fantasy and explain the effects.
5. Decide whether sexual fantasies should be kept private or shared with a partner.
6. List the categories and discuss the common types of sexual fantasies.
7. Contrast the sex differences in sexual fantasies and discuss whether there are substantial sex differences in the context of these fantasies.

PART II KEY TERMS AND NAMES TO KNOW

A. Fill in the missing word or words.

1. __________ fantasies are those in which a person returns to the same or similar visualization again and again. (245) preferential

2. __________ and __________ is a form of fantasy in which the context emphasizes the unattainable or forbidden sexual activities where the fantasizer not only programs the action but directs it as well. (247) — curiosity creativity

3. __________ or __________ is a form of fantasy in which the context is either considered as private property or to be shared with a partner. (247) — solitary shared

4. __________ is a form of fantasy in which the context recurs over and over again despite being unwanted. (248) — intruding

5. A type of sexual fantasy which involves the visualization of experiences that have never been tried in real life is called __________. (254) — experimentation

6. A type of sexual fantasy in which the concept of power is at the core is called __________. (254) — conquest

7. One of the most common types of sexual fantasy involves imagining sex with a person other than one's lover or spouse; this is called __________ __________. (255) — switching partners

8. A type of sexual fantasy that involves more than one partner at a time is called __________ __________. (256) — group sex

9. A type of sex fantasy in which a person imagines observing others engage in sex is called __________. (256) — watching

10. A(n) __________ fantasy is one in which the fantasizer visualizes him/herself as being forced into a sexual act (physically) or visualizes him/herself as the victimizer. (256-257) — rape

11. A(n) __________ __________ is a type of sexual fantasy in which a stranger is involved in near-perfect conditions and an ecstatic sexual interlude transpires. (257) — idyllic encounter

12. __________ is a type of sexual fantasy that involves inflicting or receiving pain as a source of sexual arousal. (257) — sadomasochism

B. Match the name(s) with the study.

Name(s)	Study	Key
___ 1. Nancy Friday (256-257)	a. switching partners	Crepault and Couture
___ 2. Hariton and Singer (250)	b. masturbation fantasy	Kinsey
___ 3. Crepault and Couture (255)	c. rape fantasy	Friday
___ 4. Morton Hunt (257-258)	d. fantasies of married women during coitus with spouses	Hariton and Singer
___ 5. Alfred Kinsey (258)	e. Playboy survey	Hunt

PART III SELF-TESTING--A PROGRAMMED APPROACH

1. Sexual fantasies have been regarded as deviant mainly because many psychoanalysts
   a. viewed a thought as equivalent to an act, therefore a desire to commit a deed was as sinful as the commission of it (Go to #2)
   b. thought fantasies blocked mature sexual development (Go to #3)
   c. considered fantasies to be forerunners of "deviant sexual behavior" (Go to #4)
   d. considered fantasies as recreative rather than procreative sex (Go to #5)

2. The view that a sinful thought was equivalent to a sinful deed was dogma in some religions. It was not a pervasive psychological or psychiatric view. You are incorrect. (Go to #4)

3. Psychoanalysts viewed sexual fantasies as deviant only if the fantasies portrayed something other than heterosexual acts that led to coitus. You are incorrect. (Go to #4)

4. Psychoanalysts were the only group until fairly recently to study fantasy in any depth. Many of them believed that sexual fantasies were the early signs of deviant sexual behavior. You are correct. (Go to #6)

5. Procreation was a concern of the clergy, not of psychoanalysts. Religion may have influenced their ideas and thereby contributed to their view that sexual fantasies which depicted anything other than heterosexual coitus were "deviant." You are incorrect. (Go to #4)

6. Sexual fantasies occur in a wide variety of circumstances. The commonest are those that the person finds pleasing, comfortable, and often sexually arousing and which the fantasizer returns to over and over again due in part to the fact that the fantasizer
   a. plays a central role in the story line (Go to #7)
   b. needs to share it with someone else (Go to #8)
   c. feels guilt or conflict over (Go to #9)
   d. has never experienced the circumstance in real life (Go to #10)

7. The fantasizer almost always occupies a central role in the preferential pattern fantasy. It is the one where the person prefers using this fantasy, hence repeats it again and again. You are correct. (Go to #11)

8. There are circumstances in which the person must decide whether to keep the fantasy private or share it. The decision to share or not is seldom dependent upon the fantasy's preferential nature, but on the benefits and risks associated with each alternative. You are incorrect. (Go to #7)

9. Guilt, inner turmoil, or conflict usually are produced by unwanted or intruding fantasies and are the antithesis of the preferential pattern. You are incorrect. (Go to #7)

10. Preferential patterns involve fantasies which may have been experienced previously or those which represent entirely new and untried behaviors. You are incorrect. (Go to #7)

11. Sexual fantasies serve many functions. One of the most common is to enhance both the psychological and physiological sides of sexual response. This is most often achieved by sexual fantasies that
    a. provide a safe, protective environment for engaging in made-up behaviors (Go to #12)
    b. induce or enhance sexual arousal (Go to #13)
    c. release anxiety or guilt (Go to #14)
    d. provide a means to preview an anticipated experience (Go to #15)

12. Safety with excitement is an important and common function. It does allow our imagination and sexual feelings to roam, and it is private and fictional. The erotic value of our fantasies is thereby improved. However, it is not central to enhancing both sides of sexual response. You are incorrect. (Go to #13)

13. Sexual fantasies that enhance sexual arousal by implication also enhance sexual response. The use of fantasy provides an initial boost to sexual excitement and can, for many people, move them from a plateau phase to orgasm. You are correct. (Go to #16)

14. Fantasies serve as psychological safety-valves that discharge inner tensions or needs in a relatively painless way. Fantasies in this sense can serve as a means to deal with our sexual conflicts or confusion. They are not, however, central to the enhancement of the emotional and physical aspects of sexual response. You are incorrect. (Go to #13)

15. Previewing an expected situation before it occurs through the use of fantasy serves to prepare us for what to expect and how to act. It also provides us with an opportunity to avoid potential problems by rehearsing the situation several times over. It can also test out effective ways to deal with the problems or to minimize their difficulty. But it does not enhance our sexual response. You are incorrect. (Go to #13)

16. The type of sexual fantasy in which a person is being forced or seduced into sexual acts by non-physical coercion is the flip-side of the role in which the fantasizer does the commanding. This type of sexual fantasy is often catered to in rather sexually explicit classified ads. It is a common type of sexual fantasy labelled
    a. experimentation (Go to #17)
    b. rape (Go to #18)
    c. sadomasochism (Go to #19)
    d. conquest (Go to #20)

17. Experimentation fantasy is the type wherein the fantasizer visualizes experiences that have never been tried in real life. The content usually focuses on forbidden behaviors or the unique or bizarre. It is generally a voluntary unforced action. You are incorrect. (Go to #2)

18. Rape fantasy often serves to absolve the fantasizer from responsibility of the sexual act and of culpability for enjoying it. It focuses on physical force or the threat of it and is therefore close to but not considered "non-physical" coercion. You are incorrect. (Go to #20)

19. Sadomasochism fantasy involves themes in which pain is the source of sexual arousal. These topics include visualizations of being tied, beaten, whipped, spanked, etc., or of doing the victimization. It does not necessarily involve non-physical coercion, although elements of the two may be combined (e.g., being ordered by a slave-owner to be tied and whipped). You are incorrect. (Go to #20)

20. At the core of all conquest fantasies is power; the power to command others by non-physical means to engage in sexual relations or to be commanded. You are correct.

PART IV REVIEW QUIZ

A. True or False

___ 1. Fantasies usually mean that the fantasizer wishes to engage in the visualized behavior.

___ 2. Fantasy provides a person with the opportunity to create a dimension to his or her sexual experience that is relatively unattainable in real life.

___ 3. People who insist on keeping fantasies private are immature and emotionally unready for an intimate sexual relationship.

___ 4. Sharing sexual fantasies with a partner will improve the relationship.

___ 5. Sexual fantasies can provide a safe, protected environment for allowing our sexual feelings to roam.

___ 6. Fantasy is a subtle way to express an actual desire to experience or participate in a non-sanctioned sexual activity.

___ 7. Many homosexuals have fantasies about heterosexual encounters and vice versa.

___ 8. Most people who act out their fantasies find them a disappointment.

___ 9. Few people fantasize about a different partner during sex with their lover or spouse.

___ 10. Men and women differ significantly in their sexual fantasy patterns.

B. Multiple Choice--Select the Best Answer

___ 11. The group of professionals who were the primary investigators of fantasy in any depth for over half a century were
a. psychologists
b. psychoanalysts
c. sexologists
d. physicians

___ 12. The primary fascination with a preferential fantasy lies in its
a. recurring nature
b. pleasing effect
c. sexual arousal
d. familiar theme

___ 13. Sharing fantasies may have disadvantages, such as
a. giving a distorted view of a person's preferences
b. communicating desire to act out the fantasy
c. turn-on value of fantasy fades
d. all of the above

___ 14. Sexual fantasies which are combined with masturbation are generally used to
a. counteract boredom
b. induce or enhance sexual arousal
c. boost self-image
d. relieve personal accountability

___ 15. Providing a way to preview an anticipated experience in order to prepare for what to expect and how to act is a fantasy function referred to as
a. inducing arousal
b. safety with excitement
c. controlled rehearsal
d. releasing anxiety

___ 16. In an ongoing study of sexual fantasies at the Masters and Johnson Institute, one difference that was noted between women and men was
a. most women have an interest in acting out their sexual fantasies which portray unusual sex practices, but men do not
b. most men have an interest in acting out their sexual fantasies which portray unusual sex practices, but women do not
c. men and women are equally interested in acting out their sexual fantasies which portray unusual sex practices
d. men and women express no interest in acting out their sexual fantasies which portray unusual sex practices

___ 17. A study of the sexual fantasies of married women during intercourse with their husbands by Hariton and Singer stressed that fantasy content indicated which of the following conditions?
a. Sexual problems
b. Psychological problems
c. Personality flaws
d. None of these conditions

___ 18. Reliable statistics on how many people act out their sexual fantasies in real life
a. show that the majority of men and a minority of women act out their fantasies
b. show that the majority of women and a minority of men act out their fantasies
c. show that few men and women act out their fantasies
d. are not available

___ 19. Sexual fantasies that are tried in real life usually turn out to be
a. more exciting than in the fantasy
b. more fulfilling than in the fantasy
c. disappointing
d. incorporated as a part of one's continuing sexual life-style

___ 20. The type of fantasy that involves the visualization of experiences that have never been tried in real life is classified as
a. experimentation
b. idyllic encounter
c. conquest
d. none of the above

___ 21. The type of fantasy that involves strong overtones of romance and tranquility is classified as
a. experimentation
b. idyllic encounter
c. conquest
d. none of the above

___ 22. Differences in the frequency and variety of sexual fantasies are now believed to be
   a. that men have more variety in their sexual fantasies than women and also have a greater frequency than women
   b. that women have more variety in their sexual fantasies than men and also have a greater frequency than men
   c. that the sexual fantasies of men and women are similar with no significant difference in frequency or variety
   d. unanswerable due to insufficient data

___ 23. Sexual fantasies are considered by many sexologists to
   a. be a poor substitute for real experience
   b. permit safe rehearsals of untried behavior
   c. create sexual dysfunction if not acted upon
   d. block the release of inner tensions

___ 24. Many times, fantasies conflict with our
   a. values and beliefs
   b. partner's need for shared experiences
   c. gender identity
   d. gender role

___ 25. Sharing fantasies with a partner
   a. shows maturity
   b. is a valuable contribution to the relationship
   c. risks the erotic value of the fantasy
   d. prevents sexual problems later on in the relationship

PART V CLARIFYING YOUR VALUES

Many people feel that a sexual fantasy is an expression of an actual desire to participate in or experience a given situation. Masters and Johnson have demonstrated that most people with recurrent sexual fantasies feel neither the desire nor the need to act on them in real life.

Sometimes our sexual values and our sexual fantasies seem to be in conflict, or on a collision course. The exercise that follows is designed to provide you with an opportunity to juxtapose your values about sexual fantasy. Hopefully, it may help you steer a safer course by recognizing conflicts. Indicate your degree of agreement or disagreement with the following statements by circling the appropriate response.

SA = Strongly Agree
AS = Agree Somewhat
UN = Undecided
DS = Disagree Somewhat
SD = Strongly Disagree

VALUES ABOUT SEXUAL FANTASY

	Statements about Sexual Fantasy	Degree of Agreement				
1.	A thought is not equivalent to an act.	SA	AS	UN	DS	SD
2.	A person who has "immoral" sexual daydreams or desires is as sinful as a person who acts upon them.	SA	AS	UN	DS	SD
3.	Any fantasy that portrays anything other than heterosexual acts that lead to coitus is an immature or deviant expression of the sex drive.	SA	AS	UN	DS	SD
4.	Sexual fantasy that provokes sexual desire should be stopped immediately and thoughts shifted to other things.	SA	AS	UN	DS	SD
5.	Sexual fantasy is necessary for sexual arousal	SA	AS	UN	DS	SD
6.	Sexual fantasies shouldn't necessarily be shared between sexual partners.	SA	AS	UN	DS	SD
7.	A sexual partner should be willing to play out the fantasy of the other partner.	SA	AS	UN	DS	SD
8.	Sexual fantasies that are unpleasant and unwanted and that produce stress when they recur, could benefit by counseling.	SA	AS	UN	DS	SD
9.	Sexual fantasies can serve to boost self-confidence.	SA	AS	UN	DS	SD
10.	Sexual fantasies can increase sexual excitement.	SA	AS	UN	DS	SD
11.	Sexual fantasies provide a safety valve for pent-up feelings and discharge inner tensions.	SA	AS	UN	DS	SD
12.	Sexual fantasies combined with masturbation provide a source of turn-on when a partner is unavailable.	SA	AS	UN	DS	SD
13.	Sexual fantasies that occur while making love with someone else can enhance the sexual response level.	SA	AS	UN	DS	SD
14.	Sexual fantasies allow the fantasizer to direct the action of the script and the key players.	SA	AS	UN	DS	SD
15.	Sexual fantasies are an effective means to rehearse for an anticipated sexual encounter.	SA	AS	UN	DS	SD
16.	Sexual fantasies express an actual desire to participate in the situation or act out the fantasy in real life.	SA	AS	UN	DS	SD

17. Our sexual fantasies are a reflection of our sexual values. SA AS UN DS SD

18. People with sexual fantasies that involve physical or nonphysical force may be prospective rapists or sadomasochists. SA AS UN DS SD

19. Sexual fantasies of extrarelational or extramarital sex result in guilt feelings. SA AS UN DS SD

20. Women who fantasize about rape are really yearning for such an event to occur. SA AS UN DS SD

Scoring

Questions 1, 6, 8, 9, 10, 11, 12, 13, 14, 15 are scored
SA = 1, AS = 2, UN = 3, DS = 4, SD = 5 Subtotal ________

Questions 2, 3, 4, 5, 7, 16, 17, 18, 19, 20 are scored
SA = 5, AS = 4, UN = 3, DS = 2, SD = 1 Subtotal ________

TOTAL ________

Evaluation

If your score is below 50, you probably will experience little conflict; if your score is between 51 and 69, you're pretty much in the neutral area; if your score is 70 or above, you might want to think about the probability of some conflict between fantasies and values.

PART VI ANSWERS TO REVIEW QUIZ

1. False. See text p. 252.
2. True. See text p. 246.
3. False. See text p. 247.
4. False. See text pp. 247-248.
5. True. See text p. 251.
6. False. See text p. 252.
7. True. See text p. 252.
8. True. See text p. 253.
9. False. See text p. 255.
10. False. See text p. 258.
11. (b) See text pp. 244-245.
12. (c) See text p. 245.
13. (d) See text pp. 247-248.
14. (b) See text p. 250.
15. (c) See text p. 251.
16. (b) See text p. 252.
17. (d) See text p. 252.
18. (d) See text p. 253.
19. (c) See text p. 253.
20. (a) See text p. 254.
21. (b) See text p. 257.
22. (c) See text p. 258.
23. (b) See text p. 251.
24. (a) See text p. 253.
25. (c) See text p. 248.

PART THREE / BEHAVIORAL PERSPECTIVES

11
Solitary Sexual Behavior

INTRODUCTION

This chapter examines the aspects of sexual behavior without partners and discusses topics including masturbation, sexual arousal during sleep, and the use of erotic materials.

PART I LEARNING OBJECTIVES

At the conclusion of this chapter, you should be able to:

1. Define masturbation and explain the origins of the word.
2. Contrast the early cultural, religious, and medical views about masturbation.
3. Interpret the contemporary attitudes about masturbation.
4. Describe the common patterns of masturbation.
5. List the possible reasons for the reported increase in female masturbation.
6. Compare the advantages and disadvantages of using an electric vibrator as a source of sexual stimulation.
7. Analyze the process of sexual arousal during sleep and identify its most typical forms.
8. Discuss the use of erotic materials for solitary sexual arousal and describe the four primary reasons for the use of erotica.
9. Explain the relationship between the effects of erotica and sexual behavior.

PART II IMPORTANT TERMS AND NAMES TO KNOW

Fill in the missing word, words, and names.

1. Solitary sex is often called __________ activity. (263)   autoerotic

2. Sexual self-pleasuring that involves some form of direct physical stimulation is called __________. (264) masturbation

3. The Swiss physician who is credited with labelling sexual self-stimulation as an illness was __________. (265) Tissot

4. An early American physician (one of the signers of the Declaration of Independence) who advanced the notion that masturbation caused insanity was __________ __________. (266) Benjamin Rush

5. __________ __________ is the term used to label the male orgasm during sleep. (276) nocturnal ejaculation

6. Sexually explicit material is called __________. (277) erotica

PART III SELF-TESTING--A PROGRAMMED APPROACH

1. Negative attitudes toward masturbation historically developed from several sources. The recent shift in American attitudes toward greater acceptance of masturbation is probably due mainly to
   a. 18th- and 19th-century notions about masturbation as a cause of insanity experiencing a resurgence within the moral majority (Go to #2)
   b. religious viewpoints labelling masturbation as a sin (Go to #3)
   c. medical and public opinion based on research rather than on speculation (Go to #4)
   d. recent studies that found a high prevalence of masturbatory behavior in the population (Go to #5)

2. The early notions linking insanity to masturbation have been discarded for the most part. Even those who persist in the belief would not be inclined toward acceptance of the behavior. You are incorrect. (Go to #4)

3. Some religions still subscribe to the view that masturbation is an intrinsically impure or unnatural act. This has obviously not contributed to a liberalization of attitudes toward masturbation. You are incorrect. (Go to #4)

4. By the middle of the 20th century medical authorities began to rely on the results of research instead of speculation and slowly altered their view that masturbation caused mental and/or physical illness. Public and professional opinion had shifted significantly to a more accepting attitude toward masturbation. You are correct. (Go to #6)

5. Most of the studies conducted during the past 15 years indicate that attitudes toward masturbation have relaxed considerably compared to earlier times. At the time of the Kinsey reports, both public and professional attitudes about masturbation had begun to shift. So the studies could not have contributed to the shift in attitude but were a reflection of it. You are incorrect. (Go to #4)

6. Studies on the techniques of masturbation support which of the following findings?
   a. Men and women have similar timing and tempo to their masturbatory technique. (Go to #7)
   b. Women masturbate in basically the same way as each other. (Go to #8)
   c. Men have less diversity in their masturbation patterns than women. (Go to #9)
   d. Women generally stimulate the cliteral glans directly during masturbation. (Go to #10)

7. Men and women differ considerably from each other in sexual self-pleasuring. Women tend to have greater variance in timing and tempo than men. You are incorrect. (Go to #9)

8. Women have great diversity in masturbatory technique. Masters and Johnson reported that no two women that they studied masturbated in exactly the same way. You are incorrect. (Go to #9)

9. Men in general have less diversity and more "sameness" in their masturbatory techniques. This is true despite the widely advertised gadgets to assist in male masturbation. You are correct. (Go to #11)

10. Women have a much greater variety in technique than men; however, most women avoid direct stimulation of the clitoral glans because of its high sensitivity. You are incorrect. (Go to #9)

11. The increase in the reported incidence of female masturbation may be attributed to
    a. an awareness that sexuality is a positive aspect of being female (Go to #12)
    b. women marrying at a later age and being more likely to turn to self-stimulation (Go to #13)
    c. the change in women's attire to a point where they are less sexually inhibited about their bodies (Go to #14)
    d. more women working outside of the home who are more likely to discover the masturbatory practices of other women (Go to #15)

12. The media, the Women's Movement, and sexologists have recently emphasized that females are entitled to their sexuality and that it is an important and positive aspect of being female. Women's consciousness has been raised to a point where they feel less guilty or ashamed of acting on their sexual feelings. You are correct. (Go to #16)

13. Postponement of marriage for career and/or education provides women with additional sexual options. The delay, however, would be meaningless without an attitudinal shift toward less guilt and shame about their sexual feelings. You are incorrect. (Go to #12)

14. Incidence of masturbation has not been shown to be causally related to clothing, fashion, or even nudity. The recognition and acceptance of one's sexual feelings is not a matter of choice of dress but rather a sense of oneself as being entitled to have sexual needs which may be freely acted upon. You are incorrect. (Go to #12)

15. The discovery of masturbation, especially at an earlier age, is due more to the effect of media than the fact that more women are in the labor force. Masturbation is more likely to be engaged in when a woman regards herself as deserving of sexual fulfillment from several sources (self included). You are incorrect. (Go to #12)

16. Many people show an interest in the use of erotica. The specific effect of sexual arousal that accompanies the use of sexually explicit material is achieved by
    a. the pictures or photographs (Go to #17)
    b. the printed words (Go to #18)
    c. the portrayal of sexual acts (Go to #19)
    d. the content of the material (Go to #20)

17. Pictures and photographs are styles of presentation for erotica. There are few differences in the sexual arousal induced by style. Differences that do occur are matters of preference regardless of the subject matter. You are incorrect. (Go to #20)

18. It was at one time believed that men responded more frequently and intensely to erotic readings than women did. Research shows that this is not the case. The effect produced is less dependent on the style of presentation as it is on the subject matter. You are incorrect. (Go to #20)

19. Vivid portrayal of sexual acts such as X-rated films does not differ in effect from any other style of presentation although men generally respond to style, setting, and mood of the encounter. The effect, however, is more dependent on the content, than on the style of presentation. You are incorrect. (Go to #20)

20. There appears to be no difference in the sexual effect produced by the various styles of presentation. Research evidence indicates that people are more likely to be sexually aroused by content to which they relate. You are correct.

PART IV REVIEW QUIZ

A. True or False

___ 1. Many authorities view masturbation as a normal part of sexual development.

___ 2. Masturbation is the direct, physical stimulation of the genitals.

___ 3. Sexual self-stimulation that does not lead to orgasm is not considered to be masturbation.

___ 4. Most human societies consider masturbation by adults to be an undesirable behavior.

___ 5. Traditional Judaism and Christianity differ on their view of the sinfulness of masturbation.

___ 6. Masturbation has frequently been referred to as an unnatural act by certain religions because it has no procreative goal.

___ 7. Medical opinion still considers masturbation as a contributing factor in physical and emotional illness.

___ 8. A majority of women prefer to masturbate with a vibrator.

___ 9. Current studies of sexual behavior indicate that as many women as men practice masturbation.

___ 10. The Report of the Commission on Obscenity and Pornography concluded that exposure to erotica substantially altered patterns of sexual behavior.

B. Multiple Choice--Select the Best Answer

___ 11. Solitary sexual behavior is a subject that is
a. sanctioned by the major religions
b. the major cause of guilt and anxiety
c. surrounded by misconceptions
d. practiced by a distinct minority of people

___ 12. Masturbation usually
a. begins in childhood
b. begins in adolescence
c. is terminated after marriage
d. continues in the older adult who is emotionally unstable

___ 13. The biblical reference to prohibition against masturbation known as onanism is now believed by scholars to refer to
a. non-procreative sexual behavior
b. coitus interruptus
c. nocturnal ejaculations
d. lust induced by erotic materials

___ 14. The physician who transformed masturbation from a sinful act to an illness that had to be cured was
a. Hippocrates
b. Galen
c. Paracelceus
d. Tissot

___ 15. The battle against the practice of masturbation was waged by the 19th-century medical profession through the use of which of the following methods?
   a. diet and physical exercise
   b. physical exercise and physical constraints
   c. physical constraints and diet
   d. physical exercise and surgery

___ 16. The earliest formal acknowledgment that masturbation caused no physical harm but that the worry and guilt which a child felt were the major problems of masturbation first appeared in which of the following documents?
   a. the 1935 church canon, Declaration on Sexual Ethics
   b. the 1940 pediatric textbook, Diseases of Infancy and Childhood
   c. the 1948 Kinsey report, Sexual Behavior in the Human Male
   d. the 1950 AMA report, Relationship between Masturbation and Functional Disorders

___ 17. Doubts about the healthfulness of masturbation can be attributed to which of the following studies?
   a. studies that show that nonreligious persons are frequent masturbators
   b. studies that have shown that many animals masturbate
   c. studies showing that adults who masturbate are less mature (psychologically) than those who don't
   d. none of the above

___ 18. The most common form of female masturbation involves which of the following?
   a. manually stimulating the clitoral/vulval area
   b. vibrator stimulation of the vulval/clitoral area
   c. rubbing against an object
   d. vaginal insertion

___ 19. In order to assess the health component of masturbation, it may be more helpful to
   a. count the frequency and compare it to national averages for each sex
   b. investigate whether the behavior invokes feelings of guilt or anxiety
   c. see whether other sexual outlets are being repressed or denied
   d. determine if genital injury stemming from overly vigorous or too frequent stimulation occurs

___ 20. The highest incidence and frequency of nocturnal ejaculations occurs during
   a. times when anxiety and emotional stress are high
   b. periods when other sexual activity are low
   c. the late teens
   d. none of the above

___ 21. Almost all women who report sleep-associated orgasm
   a. are oversexed
   b. masturbate
   c. get insufficient sexual satisfaction during waking hours
   d. have previously been orgasmic by other means

___ 22. Persistently disturbing sexual dreams may, in some cases,
   a. be an early sign of mental illness
   b. be ignored as a natural occurrence
   c. be a sign of underlying sexual conflict
   d. be a sign of overexposure to erotica

___ 23. Interest in reading sexually explicit materials or looking at pictures of sexual acts is
   a. a very recent practice
   b. a practice over the centuries
   c. a manifestation of certain cultures
   d. an expression of sexual frustration

___ 24. Research evidence supports the conclusion that
   a. men respond more to erotica than women
   b. women respond more to erotica than men
   c. both sexes respond to erotica in similar ways
   d. women respond psychologically and men respond physiologically to all forms of erotica

___ 25. The Report of the Commission on Obscenity and Pornography noted that
   a. most people increase masturbatory behavior when exposed to erotica
   b. most people increase coital behavior when exposed to erotica
   c. most people decrease both their masturbatory and coital behaviors when exposed to erotica
   d. most people's established patterns of sexual behavior were found to be unaltered by exposure to erotica

PART V CLARIFYING YOUR VALUES

Although the use of erotic materials (e.g., books, pictures, films, etc.) has become more accepted today than it was twenty years ago, there are still many people whose sexual value system makes them feel guilty or ashamed of this activity.

The exercise that follows is designed to help you clarify your feelings about solitary sexual behaviors. This is accomplished by placing the possible choices from the list provided on one of the steps on the ladder according to your perception of the acceptability each choice presents.

Solitary Sexual Behaviors

1. Take a course in sexual techniques that includes self-stimulation.
2. Read erotic books or magazines.
3. Masturbate while reading or looking at erotic materials (e.g., books, pictures).
4. View an X-rated film.
5. Watch animals engage in sexual activity.
6. Use a vibrator for self-stimulation.
7. Use breast stimulation as part of masturbation.
8. Insert an object into the urethral opening, anus, or vagina during or as a part of masturbation.
9. Rub genitals against an object (e.g., pillow, mattress, chair, etc.).
10. Use water massage of genital region.
11. Use a dildo or inflatable doll.
12. Use ben wa balls or suction devices.
13. Experience orgasm during sleep
14. Watch uncensored erotic cable TV.
15. Have erotic dreams.

<u>Values Ladder</u>

Most acceptable

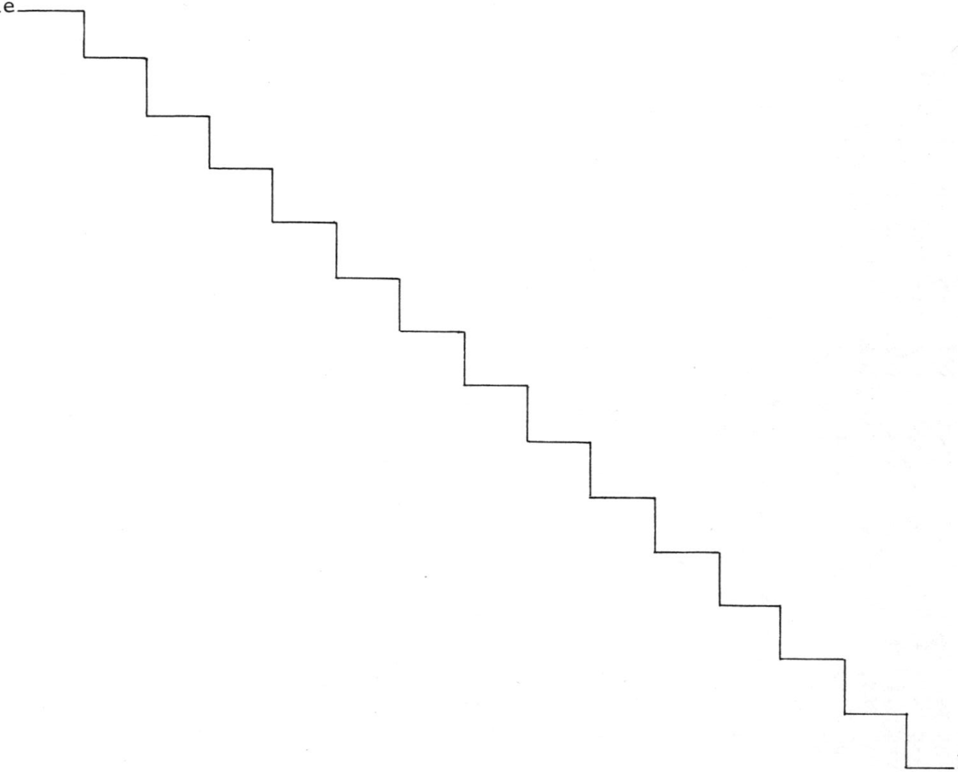

Least acceptable

Write in the number corresponding to the list of Solitary Sexual Behavior choices on each of the steps of the values ladder in order of acceptability.

Why do you think the first five choices are more acceptable to you than the last five choices (least acceptable)?

PART VI ANSWERS TO REVIEW QUIZ

1. True. See text p. 264.
2. False. See text p. 264.
3. False. See text p. 264.
4. True. See text p. 264.
5. False. See text p. 265.
6. True. See text p. 265.
7. False. See text pp. 267-268.
8. False. See text p. 269.
9. False. See text p. 274.
10. False. See text p. 278.
11. (c) See text p. 263.
12. (a) See text p. 264.
13. (b) See text p. 265.
14. (d) See text p. 265.
15. (c) See text p. 266.
16. (b) See text p. 268.
17. (d) See text pp. 268-269.
18. (a) See text p. 269.
19. (b) See text p. 275.
20. (c) See text p. 276.
21. (d) See text p. 276.
22. (c) See text pp. 276-277.
23. (b) See text p. 277.
24. (c) See text p. 278.
25. (d) See text p. 278.

12
Heterosexuality

INTRODUCTION

This chapter focuses on the most common forms of heterosexual behavior. It includes a discussion of the sexual techniques in noncoital sex play and in coitus, as well as an examination of heterosexual behavior and attitudes toward such behavior in a variety of contexts: premarital, marital, extramarital, and nonmarital.

PART I LEARNING OBJECTIVES

At the conclusion of this chapter, you should be able to:

1. Describe various techniques used in noncoital sex play.
2. Discuss the techniques of coital sex in terms of coital positions and list the advantages and disadvantages of each position.
3. Explain how stylistic variations affect coital sex including the setting, timing, and tempo.
4. Discuss the methodological shortcomings of various survey studies about sexual behaviors and attitudes.
5. Identify the changes in premarital sexual behaviors and attitudes over the past 30 years.
6. Describe the patterns of marital sex behavior in terms of coital frequency, orgasm, techniques, and satisfaction in traditional marriages and contrast these with the sexual aspects of alternative marriage styles.
7. Explain why the practice of extramarital sex is widespread today and discuss the variety of reactions people have to it.
8. Contrast consensual extramarital sex with nonconsensual extramarital sex.
9. Compare the various forms of consensual sex with each other and discuss their advantages and disadvantages.
10. Discuss the nonmarital sex options and their advantages and disadvantages and identify the factors which contribute to these practices.

PART II IMPORTANT TERMS AND NAMES TO KNOW

A. Fill in the missing word or words.

1. Stimulation of the male genitals by use of the mouth, lips, or tongue is called __________. (286) — fellatio

2. Oral stimulation of the female genitals is called __________. (286) — cunnilingus

3. __________ describes an unmarried heterosexual couple living together. (298) — cohabitation

4. Three-partner marriages are called __________. (305-306) — triads

5. __________ __________ is four or more people who genuinely regard themselves as married to each other although they do not have a legally recognized relationship. (306) — group marriage

6. Any form of sexual activity involving a married person and someone other than his or her spouse is called __________ sex. (307) — extramarital

7. When two spouses agree that one or both of them is free to engage in extramarital sex it is called __________ extramarital sex. (309) — consensual

8. __________ is a form of consensual extramarital sex where married couples exchange partners. (310) — swinging

9. When a group of people pool their resources and personal energies into emotional sharing and support that sometimes includes sexual sharing it is known as __________ __________. (312) — communal living

B. Match the name(s) with the survey.

	Name(s)	Survey	Key
___	1. Morton Hunt (295-296)	a. Two studies of human sexual behavior	Kinsey
___	2. Levin and Levin (295-296)	b. *Redbook* survey	Levin and Levin
___	3. Shere Hite (295-296)	c. *Playboy* survey	Hunt
___	4. Alfred Kinsey (296)	d. Survey of women's preferences	Hite
___	5. Constantine and Constantine (306)	e. Group marriage	Constantine and Constantine

PART III SELF-TESTING--A PROGRAMMED APPROACH

1. The most important factor in sexual technique is
   a. communication between partners (Go to #2)
   b. style of touching (Go to #3)
   c. willingness to try new behaviors (Go to #4)
   d. the setting in which the sexual encounter occurs (Go to #5)

2. When each person conveys to the other a sense of what feels good and what doesn't, the quality of the shared experience can be enhanced. The communication can be verbal, a look, a move, or some sound that clarifies preferences and feelings. It is the central ingredient in having good sex with a partner and is a very important factor in sexual technique. You are correct. (Go to #6)

3. The style of touching will vary with each individual. A touch that is arousing to one person may be uncomfortable for another. Even the same person will respond differently to one style of touching depending on the state of sexual response. What makes touching pleasurable or erotic in one instance may be a turn-off in another, so touching needs guidance, which is provided by the communication between the partners. You are incorrect. (Go to #2)

4. The willingness to try new behaviors depends on several factors (relational, environmental, emotional, etc.). Sexual technique can be enhanced if new behaviors are acceptable to both partners. This message needs to be communicated before the new behaviors are explored--otherwise the expected seuxal pleasure may turn out to be an uncomfortable experience, physically and/or psychologically. You are incorrect. (Go to #2)

5. The setting in which a sexual encounter occurs can and does often affect the satisfaction of partners; however, the fact that the setting can alter the outcome needs to be communicated. Furthermore, the setting is a modifier of the sexual technique (i.e., certain techniques lend themselves to certain surroundings: behavior will differ in a private home vs the back-seat of an auto). You are incorrect. (Go to #2)

6. There is probably no one ideal position for coitus. The reason for this stems from the fact that
   a. certain positions provide for ease of penile insertion (Go to #7)
   b. certain positions give a better chance of conception (Go to #8)
   c. certain positions give one or both partners greater freedom of movement (Go to #9)
   d. every position has advantages and disadvantages; each person is unique in each situation (Go to #10)

7. Penile insertion can be facilitated by certain coital positions but that is seldom the central issue governing the ideal choice. Even if it were the major goal, any position may be contraindicated by other intervening factors (e.g., body weight and height, age of partner(s), etc.). You are incorrect. (Go to #10)

8. Certain coital positions do provide a better chance of conception. This, however, would usually be a concern for those who are focusing on pregnancy (i.e., achieving or preventing it). In the latter instance, it is obviously a risky choice. It is also much too limiting as a condition to influence whether or not the choice is ideal. You are incorrect. (Go to #10)

9. Certain positions do provide greater freedom to one or both partners. But this is a very narrow, focused criterion in determining the best coital position. It is surely one of the considerations, but not the measure or standard. You are incorrect. (Go to #10)

10. Every individual is a unique sexual being with personal characteristics and idiosyncracies. Every position has advantages and disadvantages. When you combine the two, you have a confounding interplay of factors. Add to this another person in the form of a sexual partner, and it is plain to see the impracticality of labelling any coital position as ideal. You are correct. (Go to #11)

11. Sex surveys indicate that there has been a sizable increase in premarital coital experience. Although there are methodological problems with these surveys, most authorities agree that premarital intercourse among young women is more widespread today than it once was and that the age at first experience is declining. What do most authorities believe to be the major cause of this change in sexual behavior?
    a. More women delay marriage until they are older (Go to #12)
    b. Fewer men expect their wives to be virgins (Go to #13)
    c. There is a shift in attitude among adults from premarital sex as wrong to a more accepting attitude if it is accompanied by affection (Go to #14)
    d. There is greater knowledge and availability of contraceptive devices today (Go to #15)

12. Marriage age has not varied markedly enough to support the conclusion that there is any association between the two or, more importantly, that there is a causal relationship. You are incorrect. (Go to #14)

13. Although there has been some greater acceptance (liberalization of consciousness) about nonvirginity and cohabitation preceding marriage, studies do not support the conclusion that this shift is caused by more men feeling comfortable about the fact that their wives entered marriage as nonvirgins. You are incorrect. (Go to #14)

14. Most authorities do support the view that the increase in female premarital sex reflects a shift in attitude toward premarital sex among adults. You are correct. (Go to #16)

15. The knowledge of contraceptive devices has increased over the past 20 years and so has their availability. Studies, however, do not show that availability and knowledge of contraceptive devices are associated with premarital sex. You are incorrect. (Go to #14)

16. Lacking thorough research, it is hard to pinpoint the cause of divorce where extramarital sex is involved. The experience of many marriage counselors indicates that an extramarital affair by itself isn't the factor that causes a marriage to break up. Which of the following factors is more typically the cause?
    a. one-night stand (Go to #17)
    b. sex with a prostitute (Go to #18)
    c. sex accompanied by emotional involvement (Go to #19)
    d. an affair with another married person (Go to #20)

17. Many married people can accept extramarital sex that is purely and directly aimed at physical pleasure on an impersonal level. You are incorrect. (Go to #19)

18. Prostitution is viewed as extramarital sex at a purely physical level and not threatening to the marital relationship. You are incorrect. (Go to #19)

19. Some people are so intensely distressed at a partner's infidelity that the event alone leads to divorce. Marriage counselors report, however, that when emotional involvement accompanies the affair, it undermines the marital relationship and seems to be at the core of the marriage breakup. You are correct.

20. Extramarital sex between married persons is usually less convenient than when one person is single. However, these affairs seem less likely to be a factor in divorce since single persons are more apt to want the married ones to divorce their spouse and marry them. In addition, married couples engaging in nonconsensual extramarital affairs are more cautious about situations that pose a threat to their respective marriages. You are incorrect. (Go to #19)

PART IV REVIEW QUIZ

A. True or False

___ 1. Touching--which includes holding and cuddling--may be more important to men than women since men received less of it during infancy.

___ 2. A typical error of judgment in noncoital sex play is that one partner desires the same kind of stimulation as the other enjoys.

___ 3. Oils that contain moderate amounts of alcohol are better for tactile stimulation as they tend to be germicidal and destroy bacteria which will collect in oily residues.

___ 4. The "woman-on-top, face-to-face" position gives the male less control over ejaculation because the female has the control over coital movements.

___ 5. Women are now playing a more active role (in both sexual interactions in general and in coital sex in particular) today than they did a generation ago.

___ 6. Sex surveys indicate that among young women, premarital intercourse is more widespread today than it was 30 years ago, and the age at first intercourse is declining.

___ 7. The frequency of marital intercourse declines with length of marriage.

___ 8. There appears to be a positive correlation between sexual satisfaction and marital satisfaction.

___ 9. Women appear to have greater difficulty adapting to group marriages than men do.

___ 10. The overall sexual pleasure from an extramarital affair is somewhat higher for men and women in general than their overall sexual pleasure in their marriages.

B. Multiple Choice--Select the Best Answer

___ 11. The type of touching that turns persons into objects--regardless of gender--is rendered as
a. hard or firm pressure
b. gentle stroking and rubbing
c. massage
d. mechanical manipulation

___ 12. Most women find the insertion of one or two fingers deep into the vagina early in genital play
a. erotic
b. arousing
c. distracting
d. painful

___ 13. One of the most important considerations for successful sexual contacts is
a. communication
b. nongenital pleasuring
c. genital stimulation
d. no inhibition about experimenting with new techniques

___ 14. The "gag-reflex" is
a. psychological
b. physiological
c. conditioned
d. all of the above

___ 15. The best chance of conception occurs in which of the following coital positions?
a. Man-on-top, face-to-face
b. Woman-on-top, face-to-face
c. Rear entry
d. Side-to-side, face-to-face

___ 16. Which of the following coital positions is recommended when there is a premature ejaculation concern?
a. Man-on-top, face-to-face
b. Woman-on-top, face-to-face
c. Rear entry
d. Side-to-side, face-to-face

___ 17. Which of the following coital positions is less strenuous for both partners?
a. Man-on-top, face-to-face
b. Woman-on-top, face-to-face
c. Rear entry
d. Side-to-side, face-to-face

___ 18. Sexual enjoyment usually relates to
a. knowledge about technique
b. attitudes toward alternatives
c. skill and proficiency in technique
d. how two people relate to one another

___ 19. The percentage of women who are orgasmic during premarital intercourse has been
a. increasing
b. decreasing
c. unchanged
d. not researched adequately

___ 20. The frequency of coitus in marriage is positively correlated with
a. educational level
b. occupational status
c. religiosity
d. none of the above

___ 21. Oral-genital sex is part of the sexual repertoire in a(n)
a. minority of married couples
b. majority of married couples
c. half of married couples
d. unknown proportion of marriages

___ 22. Despite the relatively few studies on extramarital sex, what little evidence there is seems to suggest that it is
   a. a major cause of divorce
   b. mostly the consensual type
   c. fairly widespread
   d. rare, although grossly exaggerated by the media

___ 23. Most people who engage in extramarital affairs claim that
   a. sex was getting boring with a spouse
   b. they loved their spouse at the time of the extramarital affair
   c. they were away from their spouse and were lonely
   d. it wasn't much fun

___ 24. Married women who work outside of the home have
   a. a higher likelihood of extramarital sex
   b. a lower likelihood of extramarital sex
   c. no different likelihood of extramarital sex
   d. no data available to determine likelihood of extramarital sex

___ 25. Swingers as a group tend to have
   a. less premarital experience than non-swingers
   b. fewer premarital partners than non-swingers
   c. more interest in sex than non-swingers
   d. abnormal personalities

PART V CLARIFYING YOUR VALUES

Good sex is much more a matter of feelings and attitudes than it is a matter of doing the right thing at the right time, cookbook fashion. Our feelings and attitudes modify and direct our desires and moods that are expressed in the physical interaction of heterosexual activity. The quality of the shared experience with another person is thereby shaped.

The exercise that follows is intended to help you examine and clarify your own values regarding certain types of heterosexual behavior. In the left-hand column is a list of heterosexual behaviors; the right-hand column contains the possible range of attitudes you may hold about each behavior in the left-hand column. Indicate how you feel <u>right now</u> about each behavior by placing a check (√) in the appropriate column under attitudes.

Attitudes toward Heterosexual Behavior Alternatives

Behaviors	Attitudes		
	Acceptable to me	Uncertain	Not acceptable to me
Sensual nongenital touching			
Genital touching			
Oral-genital sex			
Anal sex			
Double standard of sexual behavior			
Petting to orgasm			
Celibacy			
Nonconsensual extramarital sex			
Consensual extramarital sex			
Virginity before marriage			
One-night stands			
Quickie sex			
Swinging			
Triads			
Premarital sex			
Nonmarital sex			
Post-marital sex			
Group sex			
Group marriage			

PART VI ANSWERS TO REVIEW QUIZ

1. False. See text p. 283.
2. True. See text p. 283.
3. False. See text p. 285.
4. False. See text p. 291.
5. True. See text p. 295.
6. True. See text p. 296.
7. True. See text p. 298.
8. True. See text pp. 303-305.
9. False. See text p. 307.
10. False. See text p. 309.
11. (d) See text p. 283.
12. (c) See text p. 283.
13. (a) See text p. 283.
14. (b) See text pp. 287-288.
15. (a) See text p. 290.
16. (b) See text p. 291.
17. (d) See text pp. 293-294.
18. (d) See text p. 295.
19. (a) See text pp. 297-298.
20. (d) See text pp. 298-301.
21. (b) See text p. 302.
22. (c) See text p. 307.
23. (b) See text p. 308.
24. (a) See text p. 309.
25. (c) See text p. 311.

13
Homosexuality and Bisexuality

INTRODUCTION

This chapter presents a historical perspective of homosexuality and bisexuality and discusses some controversial issues including theories on the origins of homosexuality, psychological adjustment of homosexuals, techniques of arousal, perspectives on homosexual behavior, life in the gay world, homosexuality and the law, and bisexual lifestyle.

PART I LEARNING OBJECTIVES

At the conclusion of this chapter, you should be able to:

1. Define the terms homosexual, bisexual, and heterosexual.
2. Outline the history of homosexuality from early Jewish tradition through the present day.
3. Identify and discuss the prevalent theories on the origins of homosexuality.
4. Discuss the research studies and the conclusions formed regarding the psychological adjustment of homosexuals.
5. Describe the techniques of homosexual arousal.
6. Discuss the stereotypes assigned to homosexuality, the established facts about homosexual lifestyles, and the common aspects of homosexual behavior.
7. Describe the nature of the gay world.
8. Explain the underlying attitudes toward homosexuality that affect laws and law enforcement practices.
9. Compare and contrast bisexuality with homosexuality and heterosexuality.
10. List the types of homosexual feelings and behaviors that are included in Bell and Weinberg's typology of homosexualities.

PART II IMPORTANT TERMS AND NAMES TO KNOW

A. Fill in the missing word or words.

		Key
1.	A person with a sexual preference for partners of his or her own gender is known as a(n) __________. (316)	homosexual
2.	A person sexually attracted to both males and females is known as a(n) __________. (316)	bisexual
3.	__________ is a term used by Masters and Johnson to refer to men and women who have no preference over the gender of their sex partners and who accept or reject sexual opportunities based on their own physical needs. (336)	ambisexual
4.	__________ is obsessive hostility and fear toward homosexuals. (323)	homophobia

B. Match the name with the theory.

Name(s)	Theory	Key
___ 1. Sigmund Freud (320)	a. genetic flaws	Krafft-Ebing
___ 2. Irving Bieber (321)	b. immature state of development	Freud
___ 3. Feldman and MacCulloch (322)	c. overprotective mothers, weak fathers	Bieber
___ 4. Von Krafft-Ebing (318)	d. unpleasant heterosexual experiences	Feldman and MacCulloch
___ 5. Evelyn Hooker (322-324)	e. not a form of psychological maladjustment	Hooker
___ 6. Bell and Weinberg (328-329)	f. typology of homosexualities	Bell and Weinberg

PART III SELF-TESTING--A PROGRAMMED APPROACH

1. Homophobia is expressed in many ways in our society. The ultimate expression of the hostility and fear that many people have toward homosexuals takes the form of
   a. brutal beatings or murders of homosexuals as an attempt to rid the attacker of inherent homosexual impulses (Go to #2)
   b. ridicule by jokes or derogatory labels (Go to #3)
   c. law enforcement tactics that utilize entrapment, wire tapping, hidden cameras, and other techniques of questionable constitutionality (Go to #4)
   d. prohibition to service in both the military and the ministry (Go to #5)

2. Brutal beatings and murders are the ultimate expression of hostility and fear that many people have toward homosexuals. It is often a means to rid the attacker(s) of repressed homosexual tendencies. You are correct. (Go to #6)

3. Ridicule and derogation are typical reactions to minorities. Although degrading and dehumanizing, these behaviors are less violent than other forms used against homosexuals. You are incorrect. (Go to #2)

4. Police have resorted to the use of entrapment techniques to harass and arrest homosexuals. This practice has become less common and where it still exists, it is not of the extreme sort employed by some homophobics. You are incorrect. (Go to #2)

5. The military and the ministry (in most religions) prohibit homosexuals from service. Although this practice deprives homosexuals of some meaningful and fulfilling vocations, it does not reflect the degree of brutality that is seen in other forms of homophobia. You are incorrect. (Go to #2)

6. The cause or origin of homosexuality is believed to be
   a. genetic and hormonal factors (Go to #7)
   b. arrested stage of development (Go to #8)
   c. family factors contributing to fears of heterosexual interactions (Go to #9)
   d. unknown (Go to #10)

7. Genetic theory has been pretty much rejected. Although it has been demonstrated that certain hormonal manipulations, especially early in prenatal development, can lead to homosexual behavior patterns in animal studies, the postnatal studies have not been conclusive due to methodological problems and lack of replication. You are incorrect. (Go to #10)

8. Freud's theory of psychosexual development as applied to homosexual causality is not well grounded in empirical investigation. His views on homosexuality are unclear and are generally discarded by authorities today. You are incorrect. (Go to #10)

9. Family factors have shown mixed results when put to the test of controlled research. The present evidence simply does not support the view that homosexuality stems from improper parenting. You are incorrect. (Go to #10)

10. There is no agreement among authorities about what causes homosexuality or what causes heterosexuality for that matter. The data are incomplete and better studies with more measurable research questions are needed. You are correct. (Go to #11)

11. The major difference between the sexual techniques used by homosexual men and women and their heterosexual counterparts is
    a. their greater willingness to experiment (Go to #12)
    b. their physical approach to arousal (Go to #13)
    c. their physiological responses (Go to #14)
    d. their style of using oral-genital stimulation (Go to #15)

12. Although the sexual techniques used by homosexual men and women generally mirror the techniques of heterosexual partners, there seems to be a greater willingness to experiment on the part of homosexuals. You are correct. (Go to #16)

13. The physical approaches to sexual arousal used by homosexual men and women are very varied, but so are the approaches used by heterosexuals. You are incorrect. (Go to #12)

14. Studies have shown that the physiological responses of homosexual men and women are no different from those of their heterosexual counterparts. You are incorrect. (Go to #12)

15. There are no major differences in the techniques used for fellatio between homosexual and heterosexual couples. Although lesbians are more effective in stimulating their partners via oral-genital sex and usually show less restraint, it is not the major distinguishing difference between the sexual techniques used by homosexuals and heterosexuals. You are incorrect. (Go to #12)

16. Most people "discovered" their homosexuality by
    a. early contact as a young teenager (Go to #17)
    b. confirming their suspicion by positive responses to homosexual experiences (Go to #18)
    c. finding out that their attempts to fit the expected heterosexual mold are not comfortable (Go to #19)
    d. no single pattern fits every homosexual (Go to #20)

17. Some homosexuals discover their homosexual orientation during adolescence; however, most tend to push it aside as a passing phase. You are incorrect. (Go to #20)

18. Some homosexuals suspect that they may be a homosexual before having a same-sex sexual activity, and they confirm their suspicion by positive responses to it. However, this does not apply to the majority of homosexuals, especially lesbians. You are incorrect. (Go to #20)

19. Some homosexuals discover their homosexuality only after they spend considerable effort trying to be heterosexual and finding out it just doesn't work out. This may be more true for lesbians since a large number don't adopt this sexual orientation until after they are involved in a heterosexual

marriage. Most homosexuals, however, do discover their same-sex preference before long and elaborate attempts are made to fit into the heterosexual mold. You are incorrect. (Go to #20)

20. Although research suggests that the discovery process is most likely to occur during adolescence for males and years later for females, no single pattern holds for every homosexual. People discover their homosexuality in a variety of ways; none seem to be the rule. You are correct.

PART IV REVIEW QUIZ

A. True or False

___ 1. In 1974, the American Psychiatric Association officially decided that homosexuality was not an illness.

___ 2. The definition of homosexuality includes engaging in overt sexual activity with members of the same sex as well as a preference for them as sexual partners.

___ 3. The bisexual man or woman would be rated as a 4, 5, or 6 on the Kinsey scale.

___ 4. In ancient Greece and Rome, homosexuality was accepted as natural.

___ 5. Most bio-social scientists subscribe to the opinion that homosexuality is caused by hormonal mechanisms.

___ 6. Present evidence does not support the conclusion that homosexuality is caused by improper parenting.

___ 7. Homosexuals have higher rates of emotional instability than heterosexuals.

___ 8. Gay men are more likely than lesbians to have difficulty accepting their homosexuality.

___ 9. Most homosexuals choose to remain secretive about their homosexuality.

___ 10. There appears to be a relaxing of laws and legal procedures toward homosexuals in this country over the past 10 years.

B. Multiple Choice--Select the Best Answer

___ 11. "Homosexual" is defined by the following condition:
   a. performing an overt sexual act with a member of the same sex
   b. lacking sexual attraction toward persons of the opposite sex
   c. having a preferential sexual attraction toward persons of the same sex
   d. having experienced at least one same-sex sexual contact in adult life

___ 12. Homosexuality was accepted by which of the following groups?
a. Early Jewish Kingdom
b. Ancient Greece and Rome
c. Catholic Church
d. American Medical Association

___ 13. Homosexuality is caused by
a. biological factors
b. psychological factors
c. family patterns
d. there is no agreement about the "causes"

___ 14. Homosexual arousal techniques
a. are similar to those used by heterosexuals
b. are less restricted than those of heterosexuals
c. are more inventive than those of heterosexuals
d. produce different physiological responses from those of heterosexuals

___ 15. The most frequent form of lesbian sex is
a. manual stimulation of the breasts
b. manual stimulation of the genitals
c. oral stimulation of the breasts
d. oral stimulation of the genitals

___ 16. The most common form of gay male sexual activity is
a. manual stimulation of the genitals
b. manual stimulation of the anus
c. oral stimulation of the penis
d. anal intercourse

___ 17. The process of self-discovery of a homosexual identity usually occurs in
a. childhood for both males and females
b. adolescence for both males and females
c. adulthood for both males and females
d. adolescence for males and adulthood for females

___ 18. "Coming out" usually occurs in steps starting with telling
a. family
b. best friend
c. close friends
d. colleagues at work

___ 19. Most parents will respond in which of the following ways to finding out that their child is homosexual?
a. become emotionally upset
b. urge the child to seek therapy
c. refuse to see or speak to the gay child
d. accept the fact

___ 20. Frequency of sexual activity of homosexual males is
a. the same as for homosexual women
b. higher than that of homosexual women
c. lower than that of homosexual women
d. undeterminable due to lack of research

___ 21. The number of partners the average homosexual male encounters is
- a. about the same as for heterosexual males
- b. more than heterosexual males
- c. less than heterosexual males
- d. undeterminable due to lack of research

___ 22. Changes in the law which seem less hostile to the homosexual include
- a. making homosexual acts legal
- b. sentencing the convicted person to a reduced sentence
- c. employment and housing discrimination against homosexuals being banned
- d. allowing gay men to remain in the military services

___ 23. The bisexual and ambisexual differ in that
- a. ambisexuals prefer one gender over another
- b. bisexuals never become involved in a committed sexual relationship
- c. ambisexuals accept or reject any sexual opportunity primarily on need
- d. bisexuals have frequent sexual interactions with homosexuals

___ 24. The circumstances that seem to be conducive to bisexuality include
- a. sexual experimentation with a close friend
- b. group sex
- c. intellectual coercion
- d. all of the above

___ 25. According to Bell and Weinberg's Typology of Homosexualities, homosexuals who experience a high number of sexual partners and have few sexual problems are assigned to which of the following types in the typology?
- a. open-coupled homosexuals
- b. close-coupled homosexuals
- c. asexual homosexuals
- d. functional homosexuals

PART V CLARIFYING YOUR VALUES

Some people experience obsessive hostility and fear toward homosexuals. These feelings, although often irrational, nevertheless exist. Many people who manifest homophobic feelings do not necessarily realize that they do (at the conscious level). If you ask them how they feel about homosexuals, they will often respond, "Live and let live!"

The exercises that follow are designed to help you clarify your values about homosexuality and should identify homophobic feelings.

HOMOSEXUALITY ATTITUDES

Directions

Place a check (√) on the scale between each of the sets of bipolar adjectives that indicates your general feeling about homosexuals.

	1	2	3	4	5	
Clean						Dirty
Honest						Dishonest
Healthy						Sick
Well-adjusted						Maladjusted
Strong						Weak
Brave						Cowardly
Likable						Unlikable
Moral						Immoral
Satisfied						Frustrated
Calm						Anxious
Useful						Useless
Mature						Immature

Scoring

1. Score each scale for the value above the checkmark. Example below.

1	2	3	4	5
	√			
Clean				Dirty

This would be scored as 2.

2. Add all twelve (12) scales to calculate the total. TOTAL = __________.

Evaluation

1. Scores of 45 - 60 indicate a less tolerant attitude toward homosexuals.

2. Scores of 28 - 44 indicate a neutral attitude toward homosexuals.

3. Scores of 12 - 27 indicate a more tolerant attitude toward homosexuals.

HOMOPHOBIC SCALE

Directions

Read each statement and indicate your feelings by placing a check (√) in the appropriate YES or NO response.

		YES	NO
1.	If a homosexual sat next to me on a bus, I would get nervous	___	___
2.	If my roommate told me he/she was gay, I would move out.	___	___
3.	If my best friend told me he/she was gay, it would end our friendship.	___	___
4.	If my brother (sister) told me he (she) was gay, I would tell him (her) to get professional help.	___	___
5.	If my child told me she (he) was gay, I would insist on trying to change her (his) sexual orientation.	___	___
6.	If laws against homosexuality were repealed, the number of homosexuals would increase.	___	___
7.	I find the thought of a homosexual act disgusting.	___	___
8.	Homosexuals should be barred from holding government positions.	___	___
9.	I would be upset if a child of mine had a homosexual teacher.	___	___
10.	I would not allow a homosexual to baby-sit for my child.	___	___
11.	I would not belong to any organization which had homosexuals in its membership.	___	___
12.	Homosexuals should be locked up to protect society.	___	___

Scoring

Total the number of Yes responses; total the number of No responses. YES ___

NO ___

Evaluation

If the "Yes" total is greater than the "No" total, you tend to be more homophobic than if the "No" total was greater than the "Yes" total. The opposite would mean you are less homophobic. A score of 3 or fewer "Yeses" indicates that you are very low on homophobia, while a score of 8 or more "Yeses" incidates that you have relatively strong homophobic feelings.

PART VI ANSWERS TO REVIEW QUIZ

1. True. See text p. 315.
2. False. See text p. 316.
3. False. See text p. 316.
4. True. See text p. 317.
5. False. See text p. 320.
6. False. See text p. 321.
7. False. See text pp. 324, 328.
8. True. See text p. 330.
9. True. See text p. 332.
10. True. See text p. 335.
11. (c) See text p. 316.
12. (b) See text p. 317.
13. (d) See text p. 322.
14. (a) See text pp. 324-325.
15. (b) See text p. 325.
16. (c) See text p. 327.
17. (d) See text p. 330.
18. (b) See text p. 331.
19. (a) See text p. 332.
20. (b) See text pp. 332-333.
21. (b) See text p. 333.
22. (c) See text p. 335.
23. (c) See text p. 336.
24. (d) See text pp. 336-338.
25. (d) See text p. 328.

14

The Varieties of Sexual Behavior

INTRODUCTION

Human behavior--especially sexual behavior--is varied, complex, and defies simple schemes of classification. This chapter examines the diversity of sexual behavior that is less typical than the patterns considered in the previous three chapters. It includes the concepts of normality, labeling, and stigmatization, and discusses the sexual variations in terms of their focus, unique and distinctive characteristics, and their behavioral manifestations. In addition, this chapter reviews the legal aspects of sexual behavior by providing an overview of controversies related to the laws about behaviors that deviate from the cultural standard.

PART I LEARNING OBJECTIVES

At the conclusion of this chapter, you should be able to:

1. Discuss the complexities in establishing normality, describe labeling and stigmatization patterns, and explain why labels often lead to stigmatization.
2. Describe the continuum of sexual behavior in terms of the factors that affect the degree of normality and abnormality.
3. Define paraphilia and distinguish it from sporadic sexual experimentation.
4. Identify the major types of paraphilias and describe their characteristics.
5. Define hypersexuality and identify the labels assigned to men and women considered to be oversexed.
6. Describe celibacy and discuss its characteristics, including motivations and purposes.
7. Discuss prostitution, including its motivations, advantages, and disadvantages.
8. Outline the categories of sexual behavior that are regulated by law.

PART II IMPORTANT TERMS TO KNOW

Fill in the missing word or words.

1. Applying a generalized, descriptive word or phrase to a person or group that affects how we view each other is called __________. (341) — labeling

2. __________ refers to the negative effects produced by words or phrases that brand a person as undesirable or discredit him or her in various ways. (341) — stigmatization

3. A(n) __________ is a condition in which a person's sexual gratification is dependent on an unusual sexual experience or fantasy of it. (342) — paraphilia

4. __________ is a condition in which sexual arousal occurs principally in response to an inanimate object or body part rather than a partner. (343) — fetishism

5. A(n) __________ is an individual who repeatedly receives sexual gratification and release from anxiety by dressing in the clothing of the opposite sex. (344) — transvestite

6. A sexual variation in which a person obtains sexual gratification by witnessing the sexual acts of others or by spying on them when they are undressing or nude is called __________. (346) — voyeurism

7. A(n) __________ is a person who obtains sexual gratification by exposing the sex organs to unsuspecting strangers. (347) — exhibitionist

8. The intentional infliction of pain on another person in order to achieve sexual excitement is called __________. (349) — sadism

9. The need for experiencing pain and humiliation in order to achieve sexual gratification is called __________. (349) — masochism

10. Engaging in sexual activity with an animal is known as __________. (350) — bestiality

11. When the act or fantasy of sexual activity with animals is repeatedly preferred or is the exclusive means of obtaining sexual arousal, it is called __________. (350) — zoophilia

12. __________ is a sexual variation in which the preferred or exclusive method of achieving sexual excitement is by fantasizing or engaging in sexual activity with prepubertal children. (350) — pedophilia

13. __________ is the compulsive erotic attraction to amputations. (352) — apotemnophilia

14. When sexual excitement is derived from contact with fecal matter it is called __________. (352) — coprophilia

15. __________ is sexual arousal derived from contact with urine. (352) — urophilia

16. Sexual excitement preferentially or exclusively derived from the use of enemas is called __________. (352) — kilsmaphilia

17. Sexual arousal that results from rubbing the genitals against the body of a fully clothed person in crowded situations is called __________. (352) — frotteurism

18. Sexual arousal derived from the viewing or having sexual contact with a corpse is called __________. (352) — necrophilia

19. A person who has an extraordinarily high sex drive is considered to be __________. (352) — hypersexual

20. Compulsive sexual activity in females is called __________. (352) — nymphomania

21. Compulsive sexual activity in males is called __________. (352) — satyriasis

22. Abstention from sexual intercourse is known as __________. (355) — celibacy

23. Coitus between unmarried adults is legally known as __________. (359) — fornication

24. Sexual intercourse involving a married person with a partner other than one's spouse is called __________. (359) — adultery

25. The legal situation in which a woman is enticed into sexual intercourse by a promise of marriage is called __________. (360) — seduction

26. A(n) __________ __________ is variously defined in law but most generally refers to a person who exhibits compulsive, repetitive, and/or bizarre sexual behavior. (362) — sexual psychopath

PART III SELF-TESTING--A PROGRAMMED APPROACH

1. The difficulty in deciding whether a particular sexual behavior is normal or abnormal arises from
   a. confusing dictionary definitions of "normal" (Go to #2)
   b. cultural variations (Go to #3)
   c. the difficulty of combining sociological, psychological, biological, and statistical views into a single standard (Go to #4)
   d. conflicting value judgments among the medical and legal professions (Go to #5)

2. Most dictionary definitions of "normal" state that it is something which serves as a standard, norm, rule, or principal. The words "natural" and "regular" also appear in the definition. This suggests an accepted (culturally) pattern of behavior and is fairly consistently applied. You are incorrect. (Go to #4)

3. Most behaviors, especially sexual behaviors, vary among different cultures as well as in the same culture at different periods of time. The accepted standard within one culture at one point in time is not difficult to identify (e.g., most Americans will agree that sexual activity between an adult and a child is not normal even though a small minority may consider it to be "normal"--even "healthy"). You are incorrect. (Go to #4)

4. The complexity in establishing what's normal is due to the perspective applied since there are competing views including cultural or societal customs (rules or laws), biological (natural or healthy), psychological (functional or adjusted), and statistical (frequency or majority). You are correct. (Go to #6)

5. Defining normality is always somewhat arbitrary because it involves value judgments. This often makes it difficult to establish clearcut standards for normalcy. However, value judgments are but one variable within the complexity of perspectives. You are incorrect. (Go to #4)

6. Paraphilias are conditions in which sexual arousal and gratification is dependent upon a fantasy theme of an unusual sexual experience. Which of the following paraphilias revolves around sexual objects rather than acts?
   a. Fetishism (Go to #7)
   b. Exhibitionism (Go to #8)
   c. Sadomasochism (Go to #9)
   d. Voyeurism (Go to #10)

7. Fetishism is sexual arousal that occurs principally in response to an inanimate object such as clothing, specific materials, or body parts. You are correct. (Go to #11)

8. Exhibitionism is a repetitious act wherein a person exposes the sex organs in order to obtain sexual arousal. It does not revolve around a particular sexual object; any unsuspecting stranger will suffice. You are incorrect. (Go to #7)

9. Sadism and masochism are paraphilias in which the repeated infliction of pain is used to induce sexual excitement either on another person (sadism) or on self (masochism). The focus is on the act not on the object (i.e., it doesn't matter whether the pain is induced by a whip, chain, rope, or other device for torment--what does matter is the torment or suffering). You are incorrect. (Go to #7)

10. Voyeurism is the repeatedly preferred or exclusive means of becoming sexually aroused by watching others engage in sexual activity or by spying on them when they are undressing or nude. The paraphilia focuses on the act of watching, not on the sexual object (the other person). You are incorrect. (Go to #7)

11. Several different types of pedophiles have been identified. The most common one is
    a. the aggressive pedophile (Go to #12)
    b. the personally immature pedophile (Go to #13)
    c. the regressed pedophile (Go to #14)
    d. the frustrated pedophile (Go to #15)

12. The aggressive pedophile often has a history of antisocial behavior and will often assault the victim, causing severe physical harm. Fortunately, these pedophiles are in the minority (i.e., they are the least common type). You are incorrect. (Go to #13)

13. The personally immature pedophile is a person who has never succeeded in developing the interpersonal skills to be effective with adults. This type of pedophile is drawn to children because he or she feels in control of the situation. It is the most common type of pedophilia. You are correct. (Go to #16)

14. The regressed pedophile usually has developed strong heterosexual relationships but during some point in adulthood he or she begins to develop a sense of sexual inadequacy. Sexual contact with children is often the result of a sudden, uncontrollable urge. It is not very common. You are incorrect. (Go to #13)

15. Pedophiles have recurring sexual contacts with children. Persons who have only isolated sexual contacts with children are not pedophiles but may be expressing sexual frustration regarding their inability to secure adult sexual partners. There is no such classification as a frustrated pedophile. You are incorrect. (Go to #13)

16. The street girl and the male hustler are the most vulnerable prostitutes to arrest. The reason for this is that
    a. they are unprotected by pimps (Go to #17)
    b. they are easy targets for undercover vice squad police officers (Go to #18)
    c. they are usually picked up in the major campaigns to "wipe out prostitution" (Go to #19)
    d. the laws against prostitution are against loitering in a public place (Go to #20)

17. Most street girls have pimps who provide affection and protection, and they arrange bail and help to provide clients. Male hustlers do not use pimps. You are incorrect. (Go to #20)

18. Street girls and male hustlers are no more of a target for the vice squad than any other type of prostitute. Entrapment usually results in release of the prostitute as soon as he or she is brought before a judge due to the unconstitutionality of entrapment. Few law enforcement agencies use this ineffective technique. You are incorrect. (Go to #20)

19. There are few "wipe out prostitution" campaigns and those that are carried out are short-lived since they are usually politically motivated. Although they do result in a surge of arrests and are focused at the street girl, such efforts are not the major reason for their vulnerability. You are incorrect. (Go to #20)

20. The street girl and the male hustler must practice their "profession" by placing their "wares" in a public place in order to solicit customers. Hence, they are vulnerable to arrest because most of the laws against prostitution are directed against loitering in a public place for the purpose of

prostitution or solicitation. The call girl, the prostitute in a brothel, the call boy, or the gigolo usually do not violate these statutes. You are correct.

PART IV REVIEW QUIZ

A. True or False

___ 1. The distinction between normal and abnormal is somewhat arbitrary because it involves value judgments.

___ 2. Paraphilias are more common in women than in men.

___ 3. A fetish object is often used during masturbation and incorporated into sexual activity.

___ 4. Most transvestites have a homosexual orientation.

___ 5. The voyeur is often most sexually excited by situations where the risk of discovery is low.

___ 6. Most exhibitionists are impotent in other forms of heterosexual activity.

___ 7. It is sometimes difficult to ascertain whether a caller on the telephone is being obscene or whether he is conducting legitimate sex research by the use of a telephone survey.

___ 8. The pedophile is usually a complete stranger to the child.

___ 9. There are no health risks known to result from celibacy.

___ 10. Female prostitutes seldom have orgasm in their business contacts but are normally orgasmic in private life.

B. Multiple Choice--Select the Best Answer

___ 11. Several perspectives provide definitions for abnormal behavior. Which of the following presents a psychological view?
a. It produces a personal, subjective sense of distress or interferes with the ability to function adequately in ordinary social and occupational roles.
b. It falls outside the accepted customs and rules of society.
c. It is unnatural and unhealthy.
d. It is uncommon or rare in occurrence.

___ 12. Full blown paraphilias typically become
a. magnified turn-ons achieved by variations in ordinary sexual techniques
b. more sporadic sexual experiments
c. preoccupations of sexual fulfillment to the point of being serious distractions from other responsibilities
d. all of the above

___ 13. A paraphilia which often leads to theft of another person's personal property is
a. fetishism
b. transvestism
c. frotteurism
d. klismaphilia

___ 14. Transvestites can be distinguished from female impersonators because
a. most female impersonators are married and are masculine in everyday life, while transvestites are not
b. transvestites cross-dress less elaborately and wear less makeup than female impersonators
c. transvestites want to live as women while female impersonators are entertainers and do not want another lifestyle
d. female impersonators do not use cross-dressing as a way to release tension while transvestites do reduce tension in this manner

___ 15. Fantasizing about watching others undressing is a manifestation of
a. exhibitionism
b. voyeurism
c. frotteurism
d. coprophilia

___ 16. The peak occurrence of exhibitionism occurs
a. in adolescence
b. between 20 and 30 years of age
c. between 30 and 40 years of age
d. after age 40

___ 17. The typical exhibitionist is
a. single
b. unemployed
c. below average intelligence
d. passive and shy

___ 18. The obscene telephone caller typically
a. masturbates while talking on the phone
b. boasts about himself and describes his masturbatory action in explicit detail
c. has major difficulties in interpersonal relationships
d. exhibits all of the above

___ 19. Several surveys indicate that both men and women describe sadomasochistic activities as sexually pleasurable on an occasional basis. What percentage of men and women participate in sadomasochism according to these surveys?
a. 1 - 5%
b. 5 - 10%
c. 10 - 15%
d. 15 - 20%

___ 20. Females who engage in sexual contact with animals generally
a. do so at a higher incidence than adult males
b. have vaginal intercourse with a trained pet
c. have a household pet perform cunnilingus on them
d. masturbate a male farm animal such as a horse or donkey

___ 21. The majority of pedophiles are
a. heterosexuals
b. homosexuals
c. single males
d. likely to assault their victims and cause physical harm

___ 22. Hypersexuals are people with extraordinarily high sex drives that are insistent and persistent. A central feature of most cases studied is
a. sexual activity is an insatiable need
b. sex is impersonal with no emotional intimacy
c. despite frequent orgasms, sexual activity is seldom satisfying
d. all of the above

___ 23. The major reason for the existence and persistence of female prostitution is
a. most cultures view it as a necessary evil
b. few societies legislate against it
c. it is an easy solution to economic insecurity
d. that oversexed women can achieve satiation of high sex drives

___ 24. The male prostitute in the U.S. is generally
a. soliciting male customers
b. hired to provide the customer with an orgasm
c. selling his service to wealthy, older women
d. pursuing full-time prostitution to become financially independent in the near future

___ 25. The American Law Institute recommended abolition of laws that
a. make prostitution a crime
b. criminalize incestuous relationships
c. regulate the private sexual behavior of consenting adults
d. discriminate against homosexuals

PART V CLARIFYING YOUR VALUES

Sexual behavior and our attitudes toward it vary considerably. You have had an opportunity to read about both the common patterns of sexual behavior in the last three chapters and the less typical variations in this chapter.

The exercise that follows is an opportunity to express your attitude about specific sexual variations and your feelings about their prohibition.

Place a check (√) in the appropriate space that comes closest to expressing your present attitude toward the less typical sexual variations and your feelings toward legal sanctions.

Sexual Variations

Behaviors	Attitudes					Legal Sanctions				
	E	N	U	A	P	F	M	U	D	R
Fetishism										
Transvestism										
Voyeurism										
Exhibitionism										
Obscene telephone caller										
Sadism										
Masochism										
Bestiality										
Zoophilia										
Pedophilia										
Necrophilia										
Prostitution										

Legend:

Attitudes
E = Erotic
N = Normal
U = Undecided
A = Abnormal
P = Psychopathic

Legal Sanctions
F = Felony, long-term sentence
M = Misdemeanor, short-term sentence
U = Undecided
D = Decriminalize, require treatment not jail
R = Repeal all laws regulating sexual behavior

PART VI ANSWER TO REVIEW QUIZ

1. True. See text p. 341.
2. False. See text p. 342.
3. True. See text p. 343.
4. False. See text pp. 344, 346.
5. False. See text p. 346.
6. True. See text p. 347.
7. False. See text p. 348.
8. False. See text p. 351.
9. True. See text p. 355.
10. True. See text p. 356.
11. (a) See text p. 341.
12. (c) See text p. 343.
13. (a) See text p. 343.
14. (d) See text p. 344.
15. (b) See text p. 346.
16. (b) See text p. 347.
17. (d) See text p. 347.
18. (d) See text p. 348.
19. (b) See text p. 349.
20. (c) See text p. 350.
21. (a) See text p. 351.
22. (d) See text p. 352.
23. (c) See text p. 356.
24. (a) See text p. 358.
25. (c) See text p. 359.

15

Sexual Dysfunctions and Sex Therapy

INTRODUCTION

A problem with sexual function can be a source of anxiety and frustration that leads to general unhappiness and distress in personal relationships. This chapter describes sexual dysfunctions in two dimensions: (1) conditions in which the ordinary physical responses of sexual function are impaired; and (2) the causes of these dysfunctions. The remainder of the chapter is devoted to discussing the methods and effectiveness of sex therapy in ameliorating sexual dysfunctional problems.

PART I LEARNING OBJECTIVES

At the conclusion of this chapter, you should be able to:

1. Describe the various forms of male and female sexual dysfunction.
2. List the organic and psychosocial factors that are involved in male and female sexual dysfunction and explain their effects upon the individual and society.
3. Describe the Masters and Johnson model for treating sexual dysfunction and outline the therapy format used in treatment.
4. Explain the use of sensate focus and describe the stages of exercises utilized.
5. Describe the additional methods used as supplements to the Masters and Johnson treatment model for handling problems of erectile dysfunction, premature ejaculation, ejaculatory incompetence, vaginismus, and anorgasmia.
6. Explain other treatment approaches and compare and contrast the differences between each approach and the Masters and Johnson model.
7. Explain the problems that make evaluation of sex therapy difficult.
8. State the general guidelines recommended for minimizing the risk of falling victim to unqualified sex therapists.
9. Discuss the recommended practices and attitudes that help prevent sexual dysfunction.

10. Describe other sexual problems that do not result specifically in impairment of sexual function but can cause significant emotional distress and are a source of difficulty in all relationships where they occur.

PART II IMPORTANT TERMS AND NAMES TO KNOW

A. Fill in the missing word or words.

1.	The inability to have or maintain an erection firm enough for coitus is known as __________ __________. (368)	erectile dysfunction
2.	The inability described above is also known as __________. (368)	impotence
3.	__________ __________ __________ is a condition in which a male has never been able to have coitus because of his inability to maintain an erection firm enough. (368)	primary erectile dysfunction
4.	__________ __________ __________ is a condition in which a male has succeeded in having coitus but can no longer maintain an erection firm enough for coitus. (368)	secondary erectile dysfunction
5.	Unintentional ejaculation during noncoital play, while attempting to insert a penis into a partner, or soon after coitus begins, is called __________ __________. (369)	premature ejaculation
6.	__________ __________ is the inability to ejaculate within the vagina despite a firm erection and relatively high levels of sexual arousal. (371)	ejaculatory incompetence
7.	__________ __________ is a condition where the semen spurts backward into the urinary bladder. (371)	retrograde ejaculation
8.	__________ __________ is a condition in which ejaculation in the vagina occurs only after a lengthy time period and strenuous efforts. (371)	retarded ejaculation

9. A condition in which the male has never been able to ejaculate into the vagina is called __________ __________ __________. (371) — primary ejaculatory incompetence

10. A condition in which men who have previously been able to ejaculate intravaginally normally, lose the ability or are able to do so only infrequently is called __________ __________ __________. (371) — secondary ejaculatory incompetence

11. Painful sexual intercourse is called __________. (372) — dyspareunia

12. Involuntary spasms of the muscles around the vagina in response to attempts at penetration is a condition known as __________. (372) — vaginismus

13. __________ is an outdated term that was used to describe female sexual difficulties. (373-374) — frigidity

14. __________ __________ is a term used to describe the difficulty females experience in reaching orgasm. (374) — orgasmic dysfunction

15. The currently used synonym for the above is __________. (373-374) — anorgasmia

16. __________ __________ is the condition or category of anorgasmia in which the female has never experienced an orgasm. (374) — primary anorgasmia

17. __________ __________ is the condition or category of anorgasmia in which the female was once regularly orgasmic but no longer is. (374) — secondary anorgasmia

18. The condition in which a female has had orgasm on one or more occasions, but only under certain circumstances is called __________ __________. (374) — situational anorgasmia

19. A subcategory of situational anorgasmia in which a female is orgasmic by a variety of means but never during sexual intercourse is referred to as __________ __________. (374) — coital anorgasmia

20. __________ __________ is a condition in which a female is unable to reach orgasm except on an infrequent basis. (374) — random anorgasmia

21. __________ __________ is a condition in which a woman has an orgasm almost immediately upon penetration, loses interest in further sexual activity, and often is physically uncomfortable with further coitus. (375) — rapid orgasm

22. __________ __________ __________ is a classification of causes of sexual dysfunction in which problems in sexual excitement, arousal, or orgasm are caused by physical or medical factors. (376) — organic sexual dysfunction

23. __________ __________ __________ is a classification of causes of sexual dysfunction in which sexual problems with excitement, arousal, or orgasm are caused by psychological, interpersonal, environmental, and cultural factors. (376) — psychosocial sexual dysfunction

24. An endocrine disorder in which the improper metabolism of sugar causes erectile dysfunction is __________. (376) — diabetes

25. A treatment approach that utilizes graduated touching experiences in order to reduce anxiety and teach nonverbal communication skills is called __________ __________. (386) — sensate focus

26. A behavior therapy technique that consists of neutralizing anxiety by controlled exposure is called __________. (394) — desensitization

27. A nine-step program for helping a woman learn to be orgasmic by first masturbating to orgasm is called __________ __________. (394) — directed masturbation

28. A persistent low interest in sexual activity is known as __________ __________ __________. (381) — inhibited sexual desire

29. __________ __________ is a severe phobia (irrational fear) to sexual activity. (382) — sexual aversion

B. Match the names to the work.

	Name(s)	Work	Key
___	1. Masters and Johnson (383-385)	a. Stop-start method	Semans
___	2. Helen Kaplan (394)	b. Rational-Emotive Therapy	Ellis
___	3. Jack Annon (394-395)	c. Sensate focus	Masters and Johnson
___	4. James Semans (394)	d. Sex therapy with psychoanalytic therapy	Kaplan
___	5. Albert Ellis (395)	e. PLISSIT	Annon

PART III SELF-TESTING--A PROGRAMMED APPROACH

1. Isolated episodes of not having erections are so common among men that they appear to be almost universal in occurrence. Such an episode does not mean that a man has a sexual dysfunction but it may actually reflect
   a. advancing age (Go to #2)
   b. a temporary form of stress (Go to #3)
   c. changing hormonal levels (Go to #4)
   d. reduced need for orgasmic release (Go to #5)

2. Men typically slow down somewhat in the frequency of erections as they approach the later years of life. However, most transitory or isolated episodes of not having erections are related to physical and psychological factors of a temporary nature rather than to chronological age. You are incorrect. (Go to #3)

3. Physical and psychological stress such as being sick, tired, having over-indulged, experiencing tension, lack of privacy, etc., can produce isolated episodes of non-erection or loss of erection. You are correct. (Go to #6)

4. A cyclical pattern of hormonal levels is not typical in men although women do experience these changes. There has never been a cause and effect relationship established between temporary or isolated erectile problems in men and fluctuating hormonal levels. Erectile dysfunction, however, can result from pronounced hormone deficiencies. You are incorrect. (Go to #3)

5. Whatever physiological demand there may be for the reduction of tension created by abstention or intense, long periods of sexual arousal is usually compensated for by the body (e.g., through nocturnal ejaculation). Refractory periods experienced by males after orgasm can curtail the erection response. But temporary loss of erection is most often related to other factors. You are incorrect. (Go to #3)

6. The spectator role, which can affect men and women, is usually precipitated by
   a. fears of performance (Go to #7)
   b. watching and evaluating (Go to #8)
   c. reduced intimacy and spontaneity of the situation (Go to #9)
   d. orgasmic failure (Go to #10)

7. Fears of performance often cause one or both partners to become spectators during their sexual encounter. You are correct. (Go to #11)

8. Watching and evaluating are what people do while they are in the spectator role; they do not precede the spectatoring. You are incorrect. (Go to #7)

9. Reduced intimacy and spontaneity are produced by slipping into the spectator role because of performance fears. The combination of the reduced intimacy and spontaneity with the pre-existing fears produce a reduced capacity for physical response. You are incorrect. (Go to #7)

10. Orgasmic failure is often the end result of performance fears causing the spectator role to be adopted, which results in distraction and loss of erection or lubrication. This cycle comes full turn as the fears of performance are heightened. You are incorrect. (Go to #7)

11. Women who experience vaginismus may become very fearful of sexual activity; however, the majority of women with this dysfunction
    a. do not respond to noncoital sexual play (Go to #12)
    b. do not lubricate the vagina normally (Go to #13)
    c. have difficulty achieving orgasm (Go to #14)
    d. have normal sexual desire (Go to #15)

12. Most women with this dysfunction find noncoital sexual play pleasurable and satisfying. You are incorrect. (Go to #15)

13. Most women with this dysfunction experience normal vaginal lubrication; their problem consists of involuntary muscle spasms around the outer third of the vagina. You are incorrect. (Go to #15)

14. Surprisingly, many women with this dysfunction find that their orgasmic response is relatively unaffected by the problem. They have normal sexual arousal and are upset by their inability to enjoy coitus. You are incorrect. (Go to #15)

15. Most women whose outer third of the vagina experiences involuntary spasms in response to attempts at vaginal penetration are dismayed that their normal sexual responses are accompanied by this dysfunction. Women with vaginismus usually have normal sexual desire and are upset by their inability to share in the enjoyment of coitus with their partners. You are correct.

16. Psychosocial factors are thought to contribute to the origins of sexual dysfunction. Among the most common is poor communication, both in sexual and nonsexual areas of a relationship. Communications problems fall under the psychosocial causes in which of the following categories?
   a. developmental factors (Go to #17)
   b. personal factors (Go to #18)
   c. interpersonal factors (Go to #19)
   d. deep-seated personality factors (Go to #20)

17. Developmental factors include such things as parent-child relationships, family attitudes toward sex, traumatic childhood experiences, adolescent sexual experiences and gender identity conflicts. Communication is not a developmental factor. You are incorrect. (Go to #19)

18. Personal factors include the individual's fears and anxieties over things like pregnancy, venereal disease, rejection, loss of control, pain, intimacy, etc. Other feelings like guilt, depression, and poor self-esteem are personal factors as well. Even the lack of sexual information and blind acceptance of cultural myths are of a personal nature. Communication, however, is not as it involves another or other persons. You are incorrect. (Go to #19)

19. Poor communication is an interpersonal factor because it is a relational issue just as power struggles, hostility, distrust, deceit, and conflicts in the sex value systems of partners are relational issues. You are correct.

20. Deep-seated personality factors are no longer considered to be significant as sexologists today consider that most people with sexual dysfunctions have normal personalities, and do not exhibit mental illnesses. Before the Masters and Johnson studies were released, it was generally thought that sexual dysfunctions were due to personality anomalies. You are incorrect. (Go to #19)

PART IV REVIEW QUIZ

A. <u>True or False</u>

___ 1. Premature ejaculation is probably the most common sexual dysfunction among men in the general population.

___ 2. Ejaculatory incompetence is mainly seen in men over age 35.

___ 3. Diagnosis of vaginismus can only be made with certainty by a careful pelvic examination.

___ 4. Any woman who does not experience orgasms or who is unconcerned about how she reaches her orgasms should be encouraged to seek out sex therapy.

___ 5. It is not always possible to identify precisely the cause of a specific sexual dysfunction in a given person.

___ 6. Rapid orgasm in women has no known physical cause.

___ 7. Sexual dysfunctions are generally caused by religious beliefs which are forced upon children.

___ 8. Too much sex information is frequently the cause of many sexual dysfunctions.

___ 9. Treatment of sexual dysfunctions takes a very long time of intense therapy.

___ 10. Since poor communication is at the root of many sexual dysfunctions, sensate focus periods at the outset of treatment include as much verbal interchange as necessary to direct the touching activity.

B. Multiple Choice--Select the Best Answer

___ 11. Erectile dysfunction usually takes the form of
a. total absence of erection
b. partial erections
c. firm erections that quickly disappear
d. normal erections under some circumstances

___ 12. Masters and Johnson classified a man as secondarily impotent if
a. he was formerly having no erectile problems
b. he has erections during less than half of his sexual encounters
c. his erection problems occurred in at least 25 percent of his sexual encounters
d. erectile problems are caused by stress

___ 13. The American Psychiatric Association defines premature ejaculation
a. in terms of reasonable voluntary control
b. as ejaculation before the partner experienced orgasm in at least 50 percent of their coital episodes
c. as ejaculation within 3 minutes of vaginal intromission
d. as ejaculation before the male wanted to ejaculate

___ 14. Erectile difficulties can occur if a premature ejaculator struggles to control his sexual arousal
a. by varying sexual fantasies
b. by altering situations
c. by shortening the time of noncoital play
d. by using distractions

___ 15. Masters, Johnson, and Kolodny estimate that some _____ percent of American men have at least a moderate degree of difficulty controlling rapid ejaculation
a. 5 - 10
b. 15 - 20
c. 30 - 35
d. 40 - 45

___ 16. The opposite of premature ejaculation is
a. retrograde ejaculation
b. primary ejaculatory incompetence
c. retarded ejaculation
d. secondary ejaculatory incompetence

___ 17. Male dyspareunia is typically centered in the
a. penis
b. testes
c. prostate
d. seminal vesicles

___ 18. Females who are affected by vaginismus are generally
a. in their adolescence
b. in their early 20s
c. past the age of 35
d. of any age

___ 19. Primary anorgasmia refers to women who
a. have difficulty reaching orgasm
b. have never had an orgasm
c. were regularly orgasmic at one time but no longer are orgasmic
d. have had orgasms on one or more occasions

___ 20. It is generally estimated that organic causes are responsible for __________ percent of sexual dysfunction cases.
a. 5 - 10
b. 10 - 20
c. 20 - 30
d. 30 - 40

___ 21. Painful intercourse in males may be due to
a. inflammation or infection of the genitalia
b. irritation by the tail of an IUD
c. exposure to a vaginal contraceptive
d. all of the above

___ 22. Rigid religious upbringing seems to be a common factor in
a. secondary impotence
b. dyspareunia
c. primary anorgasmia
d. random anorgasmia

___ 23. The traditional psychoanalytic view of sexual dysfunction contends that
a. the dysfunction is not the primary problem but is instead a symptom of a deeper psychological disturbance
b. the dysfunctions reflect Oedipal and Electra type conflicts
c. old fears of childhood are reawakened by adult sexual encounters causing psychological conflict and dysfunction
d. dysfunctions are conditioned responses that are maintained by positive reinforcement

___ 24. At the beginning of therapy in the Masters and Johnson Therapy Format,
   a. couples are instructed to refrain from verbal communication
   b. couples are asked to refrain from genital contact
   c. couples are asked to refrain from touching one another
   d. couples are formally instructed about sexual anatomy and physiology

___ 25. Helen Kaplan's treatment approach differs in which of the following ways from the Masters and Johnson methods?
   a. Kaplan views human sexual response as three phases rather than four.
   b. Kaplan uses a lengthened form of sex therapy that addresses unconscious conflicts.
   c. Kaplan uses a single therapist approach rather than a co-therapy team.
   d. All of the above

PART V CLARIFYING YOUR VALUES

Results of therapy at the Masters and Johnson Institute reveal that the success rates for treating male and female sexual dysfunctions vary considerably. Given these data and the feelings you have regarding sexual dysfunction, if you or your sexual partner were sexually dysfunctional, which of the following would you seek professional help to modify? Place a check (√) under the appropriate response.

Sexual Dysfunction	Therapeutic Intervention		
	Definitely Seek Help	Uncertain	Ignore It
Male			
Primary impotence			
Secondary impotence			
Premature ejaculation			
Ejaculatory incompetence			
Dyspareunia			
Retarded ejaculation			
Retrograde ejaculation			
Female			
Primary anorgasmia			
Secondary anorgasmia			
Situational anorgasmia			
Vaginismus			
Dyspareunia			
Coital anorgasmia			
Random anorgasmia			
Rapid orgasm			

PART VI ANSWERS TO REVIEW QUIZ

1. True. See text p. 370.
2. False. See text p. 371.
3. True. See text p. 373.
4. False. See text p. 375.
5. True. See text p. 376.
6. True. See text p. 378.
7. False. See text p. 379.
8. False. See text p. 380.
9. False. See text p. 383.
10. False. See text p. 386.
11. (b) See text p. 368.
12. (c) See text p. 368.
13. (a) See text p. 369.
14. (d) See text p. 370.
15. (b) See text p. 370.
16. (c) See text p. 371.
17. (a) See text p. 372.
18. (d) See text p. 372.
19. (b) See text p. 374.
20. (b) See text p. 376.
21. (d) See text p. 378.
22. (c) See text p. 379.
23. (a) See text p. 380.
24. (b) See text p. 386.
25. (d) See text p. 394.

16

Sexual Disorders and Sexual Health

INTRODUCTION

Sexual health and total health are inextricably interrelated. Both are affected by physical and psychological factors and high or low levels of either one can alter the other. This chapter focuses on the physical factors that affect sexuality by examining the impact of illness on sexuality, the drugs that influence sexual desire and sexual functions, sexually transmitted diseases, and other infections of the sex organs.

PART I LEARNING OBJECTIVES

At the conclusion of this chapter, you should be able to:

1. Describe the direct and indirect ways that illnesses can affect sexuality.
2. Explain how diseases or injury to the nervous system can lead to sexual difficulties and identify the most common types of neurologic conditions that affect sexuality.
3. Discuss the endocrine disorders that are commonly associated with sexual problems.
4. Identify the types of heart disease that can affect sexual functioning.
5. List the types of cancer that impact on sexuality and discuss their effects on sexual functioning.
6. Describe the effect of alcoholism on sexuality and discuss the reasons why the problems develop.
7. Compare the effects of various substances, prescriptions, and nonprescription drugs on sexual desire and sexual function.
8. List the most common types of sexually transmitted diseases and identify their symptoms, diagnosis, and treatment.
9. State the ways to minimize the chances of contracting STDs and the ways to avoid spreading them.
10. Outline other common infections of the sex organs and identify their symptoms, diagnosis, and treatment.

PART II IMPORTANT TERMS TO KNOW

Fill in the missing word or words.

1. A spinal cord injury that involves paralysis of the lower limbs is called __________. (400) — paraplegia
2. A spinal cord injury that involves paralysis of all four limbs is called __________. (400) — quadriplegia
3. A disease which often affects sexual function that involves patchy damage to the protective covering of the nerves is known as __________ __________. (403) — multiple sclerosis
4. A chronic endocrine disorder that can cause nerve damage and often results in erectile dysfunction or retrograde ejaculation in men or secondary anorgasmia in women is called __________. (404) — diabetes
5. The surgical removal of the breast that is often used to treat breast cancer is called a(n) __________. (406) — mastectomy
6. Partial or total surgical removal of the uterus is called a(n) __________. (408) — hysterectomy
7. The surgical removal of the prostate gland is called a(n) __________. (408) — prostatectomy
8. A(n) __________ is a substance that increases or is believed to increase a person's sexual powers or desire. (411) — aphrodisiac
9. An illicit nervous system stimulant drug that has a street reputation as a strong sexual stimulant also known as "snow" is the drug __________. (412) — cocaine

10. An inhalant that is sometimes used to prolong or intensify orgasm is the drug __________ __________. (414) — amyl nitrate

11. Infections that are spread mainly by sexual contact are called __________ __________ __________ or STDs. (414) — sexually transmitted diseases

12. The oldest and most common form of STD, characterized in men by a discharge of pus from the urethra, is known as __________. (415, 416) — gonorrhea

13. The STD caused by a spiral-shaped microorganism is known as __________. (417) — syphilis

14. A painless sore that appears in the primary stage of syphilis is called a(n) __________. (418) — chancre

15. __________ syphilis is the stage that is marked by a sore. (418) — primary

16. __________ syphilis begins after the sore heals. (418) — secondary

17. Late syphilis is called the __________ stage. (418) — tertiary

18. Syphilis contracted by the unborn fetus from an infected mother is called __________ syphilis. (418-419) — congenital

19. A common STD that is marked by clusters of small, painful blisters on the genitals which burst after a few days and leave small ulcers that are closely related to cold sores or fever blisters is called genital __________. (419) — herpes

20. __________ __________ are parasites that invade the pubic region. (420) — pubic lice

21. Any inflammation of the male urethra that is not caused by gonorrhea is called __________ __________. (421) — nonspecific urethritis

22. Dry, usually painless nodules that grow on or near the genitals, that are caused by a virus and are sexually transmitted are called __________ __________. (421) — venereal warts

23. Vaginal inflammation from infection or chemical irritation is known as __________. (422) — vaginitis

24. __________ __________ is an infection of the vagina caused by bacteria that causes a frothy, foul-smelling discharge. (423) — trichomonas vaginitis

25. A fungus infection caused by an overgrowth of candida albicans in the vagina is called __________ __________. (423) — monilial vaginitis

26. An infection of the bladder closely related to sexual activity in women is called __________. (423) — cystitis

27. Inflammation of the prostate gland is called __________. (424) — prostatitis

PART III SELF-TESTING--A PROGRAMMED APPROACH

1. Illnesses affect sexuality in direct and indirect ways. Which of the following is an indirect effect?
   a. disruption of normal reflexes of sexual response (Go to #2)
   b. medicines that cause sexual side effects (Go to #3)
   c. effects that accompany illness such as fatigue or pain (Go to #4)
   d. belief that illness will prevent sexual function (Go to #5)

2. Spinal cord injury often causes a disruption of normal reflexes of sexual response. It has a direct effect upon sexuality. You are incorrect. (Go to #5)

3. Medicines that are used to treat many illnesses cause impairment of sexual function. Many of the medications used to treat hypertension cause sexual difficulties (e.g., Aldomet causes erectile dysfunction). It is a direct effect. You are incorrect. (Go to #5)

4. Weakness, fatigue, or pain which often arises during illness can and generally does have a direct impact upon the sick person's sexual desire and/or sexual functioning. You are incorrect. (Go to #5)

5. Mind and body are inextricably interrelated, especially in regard to sexuality. Feelings and emotions often prevent well people as well as sick people from functioning normally. These are indirect effects. You are correct. (Go to #6)

6. The neurological condition that is most likely to cause sexual difficulties is
   a. spinal cord injury (Go to #7)
   b. brain tumors (Go to #8)
   c. epilepsy (Go to #9)
   d. polio (Go to #10)

7. Injuries to the spinal cord often result in a significant loss of sexual function. You are correct. (Go to #11)

8. Tumors of the brain do not usually lead to sexual problems unless they are tumors of the pituitary or hypothalamus. You are incorrect. (Go to #7)

9. Epilepsy has little effect on sexual function although, because of a sense of inferiority, epileptics may avoid sexual opportunities in the mistaken notion that arousal will cause a seizure. You are incorrect. (Go to #7)

10. Although polio can cause spinal damage, it affects muscular function rather than sensation; therefore, people with paralysis from polio seldom experience impaired sexual functioning. You are incorrect. (Go to #7)

11. The primary factor in a decline in the capacity for sexual activity after a heart attack is due to
    a. reduced maximum oxygen uptake (Go to #12)
    b. painful muscle spasms in the chest (angina) during physical exertion (Go to #13)
    c. psychological factors, such as anxiety that sexual excitement may precipitate another heart attack (Go to #14)
    d. decreased vasocongestion capacity which results in the inability to have an erection (male) or to lubricate (female) (Go to #15)

12. Severe forms of heart attack can produce limitations in the capacity for sexual activity. Most of the studies have shown that sexual difficulties following heart attacks are common. The difficulties are not primarily due to a physical factor such as reduced max. VO_2. You are incorrect. (Go to #14)

13. Angina is commonly caused by a reduction in blood supply to the heart muscle. This is often a precursor to a heart attack as well as a result of one. Although sexual difficulties have been shown by several research studies to occur in men following a heart attack, the primary factor is not a physical one. You are incorrect. (Go to #14)

14. The primary factor that research studies have shown to be associated with sexual difficulties following a heart attack is a mental one such as anxiety. You are correct. (Go to #16)

15. Decreased vasocongestion is typically caused by psychogenic factors rather than physiological ones. Research studies have shown that the primary factor in the sexual difficulties experienced post-coronary is not a physical one but a mental one such as worry. You are incorrect. (Go to #14)

16. Certain drugs cause sexual difficulties for men and women. These include both prescription and nonprescription drugs. One drug that is commonly used to treat high blood pressure causes sexual problems for about 15 percent of the men and women who take it. This prescription drug (Aldomet) can produce
    a. retarded ejaculation in men (Go to #17)
    b. decreased libido and impaired sexual arousal in women (Go to #18)
    c. reduced vaginal lubrication (Go to #19)
    d. reduced testosterone production (Go to #20)

17. Inhibited or retarded ejaculation is one of the side effects attributed to Ismelin (guanethidine) in about half of the men who use it. Aldomet causes erectile dysfunction in about 10 to 15 percent of the men who use it. The percentage rises to almost 50 percent in high dose users. Aldomet does not cause retarded ejaculation. You are incorrect. (Go to #18)

18. Decreased libido and impaired sexual arousal has been reported to occur in about 15 percent of the women who use Aldomet for the treatment of high blood pressure. You are correct.

19. Reduced vaginal lubrication can be an indirect result of decreased libido and impaired sexual arousal; however, it is not directly caused by the use of Aldomet. Antihistamines have been shown to reduce vaginal lubrication and sometimes cause painful intercourse. You are incorrect. (Go to #18)

20. Reduced testosterone production has been shown to be caused by heavy marijuana usage. Marijuana use also has been shown to disturb sperm production. Aldomet does not affect testosterone levels. You are incorrect. (Go to #18)

PART IV REVIEW QUIZ

___ 1. Most spinal cord injured people lose their interest in sexual activity.

___ 2. Epilepsy produces a significant reduction in the ability to function sexually.

___ 3. About one-third of all diabetic women have secondary anorgasmia.

___ 4. Women who have had heart attacks seem to be less likely to develop subsequent sexual problems than men.

___ 5. Following a mastectomy, most women experience a reduction in the frequency of sexual activity.

___ 6. Following a prostatectomy for cancer, men frequently experience erectile dysfunction.

___ 7. The majority of alcoholics have sexual problems.

___ 8. There have been virtually no studies on the effects of marijuana on sexuality.

___ 9. Syphilis is the oldest and most common form of STD.

___ 10. The cure for genital herpes is twofold: (1) antibiotic ointment on the ulcers; and (2) injection of penicillin in its dormant state.

B. Multiple Choice--Select the Best Answer

___ 11. Most spinal cord injured men
a. lose the ability to have normal erections
b. lose the ability to ejaculate
c. become infertile
d. all of the above

___ 12. Women with spinal cord injuries usually
a. lose their genital sensations and orgasmic function
b. lose all vaginal lubrication
c. become infertile
d. do not experience serious sexual problems

___ 13. Persons with brain tumors usually
a. lose their sexual drives
b. lose their ability to function sexually
c. become infertile
d. do not experience serious sexual problems

___ 14. The primary cause of sexual problems in both diabetic men and women is
a. circulatory problems
b. a form of nerve damage
c. the effect of insulin injections
d. of psychogenic origin

___ 15. The major cause of sexual problems in post-coronary patients is
a. anti-clotting medications
b. circulatory inefficiency
c. of psychogenic origin
d. reduced capacity for physical exertion

___ 16. The best time for a breast self-examination is
a. right before the woman's expected menstrual period
b. during the menstrual period
c. after the menstrual period is over
d. any day of the month just as long as it is the same day every month

___ 17. Removal of a breast can create
a. rejection by spouse
b. concerns about physical attractiveness
c. reduced frequency of sexual activity
d. all of the above

___ 18. On the average, how many years does it take for CIS to progress to true cancer (ICC)?
a. 2 years
b. 4 years
c. 6 years
d. 8 years

___ 19. The only "foolproof" way of diagnosing cancer of the uterus is a
a. Pap smear
b. D&C
c. hysterectomy
d. all of the above

___ 20. Treatment for cancer of the prostate consists of
a. prostatectomy
b. radiation therapy
c. hormone therapy
d. any or all of the above

___ 21. Cancer of the testis is a relatively rare condition that is most common
a. in the 20s and 30s
b. between 40 and 60 years of age
c. after the age of 60 years
d. at no particular age

___ 22. Alcoholism is usually accompanied by sexual problems because
a. it directly affects hormone production
b. it directly affects circulatory function
c. it directly affects libido
d. all of the above

___ 23. Which of the following drugs is used to prolong or intensify the sensation of orgasm?
a. alcohol
b. LSD
c. amyl nitrate
d. marijuana

___ 24. A yellowish discharge from the tip of the penis and painful, frequent urination are the first indications of
a. gonorrhea
b. syphilis
c. genital herpes
d. granuloma inguinale

___ 25. Disagreeable odors emanating from the vagina often accompany vaginal infections. Which of the following is caused by a type of fungus or yeast infection?
a. trichomonas vaginitis
b. monilial vaginitis
c. hemophilus vaginalis
d. cystitis

PART V CLARIFYING YOUR VALUES

Sexual health and total health are not only interrelated and interdependent but depend on freedom from physical and emotional limitations. A component of the emotional dimension is our own value system on which our choices about how to live our lives are made.

Our values play an important role in our choices regarding sexual health. The exercise that follows is intended to raise some important questions about decisions and actions you may face in life situations now and in the future.

VALUES CHOICES

Complete each of the following sentences by placing a rank number (1, 2, 3, 4) to signify the order assigned to each of the four choices following each unfinished sentence.

	RANK
1. The worst thing that I could find out about my sexual health is that I . . .	
a. developed a neurologic condition that could impair my sexual functioning	____
b. developed an endocrine disorder that could impair my sexual functioning	____
c. developed a chronic disease that could impair my sexual functioning	____
d. developed a sexually transmitted disease	____
2. If I thought that I had contracted an STD, I would . . .	
a. try to treat it myself	____
b. go to my family physician for diagnosis and treatment	____
c. wait to see if more symptoms developed	____
d. tell my sexual partner(s) about it as soon as it was confirmed	____
3. If my sexual partner(s) contracted genital herpes, I would . . .	
a. never have sex with him/her/them again	____
b. think he/she/they was/were having sex with someone else	____
c. think I gave it to him/her/them	____
d. be confused and angry and not know what I'd do	____
4. The worst thing that I could find out about my mate is that he/she . . .	
a. is sterile	____
b. has an STD	____
c. is promiscuous	____
d. is using an aphrodisiac	____

5. The best way to prevent getting a STD for me would be to . . .
   a. practice abstinence ____
   b. have as few sexual partners as possible ____
   c. use a condom and a chemical contraceptive ____
   d. ask my partner if he/she has an STD ____

What factor(s) do you think contributed to your choices? List them under the categories below.

1. (Sexual health)

2. (STD)

3. (Genital herpes)

4. (About mate)

5. (Prevention)

PART VI ANSWERS TO REVIEW QUIZ

1. False. See text p. 403.
2. False. See text p. 403.
3. True. See text p. 404.
4. True. See text p. 404.
5. True. See text p. 406.
6. True. See text p. 408.
7. True. See text pp. 408-411.
8. False. See text pp. 412-414.
9. False. See text p. 415.
10. False. See text p. 420.
11. (d) See text p. 403.
12. (a) See text p. 403.
13. (d) See text p. 403.
14. (b) See text p. 404.
15. (c) See text p. 404.
16. (c) See text p. 405.
17. (d) See text p. 406.
18. (d) See text p. 406.
19. (b) See text pp. 407-408.
20. (d) See text p. 408.
21. (a) See text p. 408.
22. (a) See text p. 411.
23. (c) See text p. 414.
24. (a) See text p. 416.
25. (b) See text p. 423.

17

Coercive Sex: The Varieties of Sexual Assault

INTRODUCTION

This chapter examines the historical, legal, social, and psychological perspectives about coercive sex. It focuses on rape, incest, sexual harassment at work, and sex victimology.

PART I LEARNING OBJECTIVES

At the conclusion of this chapter, you should be able to:

1. State the legal definition of rape and incest.
2. Describe the early laws against rape and the myths about rape.
3. Identify the patterns of rape.
4. Explain the legal considerations facing rape victims.
5. State the phases of the aftermath of rape.
6. Outline the general characteristics of convicted rapists and discuss their patterns of rape.
7. Identify the common myths about incest and state the facts that override these myths.
8. Discuss the various patterns of incest and the research findings about the effects of incest on its victims.
9. Identify the situations in which sexual harassment occurs.
10. Discuss the cultural and societal attitudes and practices that foster sex victimology.

PART II IMPORTANT TERMS TO KNOW

Fill in the missing word or words.

1. The need to have another person's testimony to confirm that a rape occurred is called __________. (429) corroboration

2. The most common form of rape in which penile penetration of the vagina is achieved by force or threat of force is called __________ rape. (429) forcible

3. The type of sexual assault in which one person rapes another is called __________ rape. (430) solo

4. The type of sexual assault in which several people take turns raping a victim is called __________ rape. (430) gang

5. __________ rape is a subcategory of forcible rape in which a person is forced into unwanted sexual activity on a date or at a party. (430) date

6. __________ rape is a subcategory of forcible rape in which one spouse forces the other spouse into unwanted sexual activity. (430) mate

7. Sexual intercourse with a girl below the legal age of consent is known as __________ rape. (430) statutory

8. The type of forcible rape in which the rapist intimidates the victim by using a weapon, physical force, and threats of bodily harm is called __________ rape. (436) power

9. The type of forcible rape in which the rapist brutalizes the victim and expresses rage and hatred by physical assault and verbal abuse is called __________ rape. (436) anger

10. The type of forcible rape in which sexuality and aggression are fused together and the suffering of the victim is the primary source of the rapist's satisfaction is called __________ rape. (436) — sadistic

11. __________ is a term that refers to sexual acts between close relatives. (437) — incest

12. __________ __________ is the recent variety of sexual abuse using children in the production of pornographic photographs, movies, or videotapes. (439) — child pornography

PART III SELF-TESTING--A PROGRAMMED APPROACH

1. Laws concerning rape changed dramatically over the centuries. In particular, the last decade has seen a significant change in public awareness of rape. A major influence in this "raised consciousness" about rape occurred mainly through the activities of
   a. State Legislatures (Go to #2)
   b. the U.S. Supreme Court (Go to #3)
   c. the Women's Movement (Go to #4)
   d. the American Civil Liberties Union (Go to #5)

2. Many states have enacted legislation that prevents a rape victim's past sexual behavior from being introduced into the trial by a defense attorney. However, this advance has probably been due to the lobbying activities and public education programs of concerned pressure groups. You are incorrect. (Go to #4)

3. The U.S. Supreme Court hears cases that test the constitutionality of laws and lower court decisions. The Court has not contributed to the public's consciousness about rape. You are incorrect. (Go to #4)

4. The Women's Movement has been the force behind the increase in public awareness and consciousness about rape. Women have raised the major issues and have demanded improvement in services to rape victims. You are correct. (Go to #6)

5. The American Civil Liberties Union has done much to protect the constitutional rights of all people including the rights of victims as well as the rights of those who violate them. They have not, however, played a major role in raising the level of public awareness or consciousness about rape. You are incorrect. (Go to #4)

6. There are many myths about rape and about rapists. Which of the following statements is not a myth?
   a. Most women secretly "want" to be raped. (Go to #7)
   b. Most women precipitate rape by enticing or seducing the assailant with incautious and provocative behavior. (Go to #8)
   c. Rapes are committed by oversexed men. (Go to #9)
   d. Most rapes are acts of violence rather than acts of passion. (Go to #10)

7. Although many women may fantasize about being raped, they do not indicate real-life sexual desire. You are incorrect. (Go to #10)

8. The popular belief that women who are raped instigated the act by some form of "provocation" is invalidated by the fact that many rape victims are elderly women and young children. You are incorrect. (Go to #10)

9. The view that rapists are oversexed is unsupported in the studies conducted on convicted rapists. Most rapists do not lack sexual partners. One study found that none of the rape cases included in the research showed sex as the dominant motive; rather, rape was an expression of power or anger and not an act of sexual desire. You are incorrect. (Go to #10)

10. Studies conducted on convicted rapists report that the act of rape is predominantly an aggressive one, a way to reassure the rapist about his strength and identity and as a means of punishment or revenge. Rape is seldom an act of passion. You are correct. (Go to #11)

11. Research on incest has a number of limitations due in large part to sampling problems. One distortion that this has introduced is the notion that the most frequent pattern of incest is
    a. mother-son (Go to #12)
    b. father-daughter (Go to #13)
    c. brother-sister (Go to #14)
    d. parent-child of same gender (Go to #15)

12. Mother-son incest is rare. One or both parties to this type of incest is usually psychologically disturbed. You are incorrect. (Go to #15)

13. Father-daughter incest is often viewed as the most common pattern since it is most typically reported or brought to treatment. In reality, it is not the most common pattern and therefore a distortion of the fact. You are correct. (Go to #16)

14. Sibling incest is almost never reported or brought to treatment; therefore, it seems to be far less common than father-daughter incest. Several surveys have found that brother-sister incest is the most frequent pattern. You are incorrect. (Go to #13)

15. Parent-child of same gender incest is exceptionally rare. Father-son incest accounts for less than 1 percent of all incest cases and mother-daughter incest seems to be the rarest form of nuclear family sex. You are incorrect. (Go to #13)

16. Sexual harassment at work appears in a number of different forms. The most typical situation occurs when
   a. a boss or supervisor makes sexual compliance a condition for keeping a job, getting a promotion, or obtaining work-related benefits (Go to #17)
   b. a prospective employer makes it clear that hiring depends on sexual availability (Go to #18)
   c. the employee is subjected to indirect but less than subtle sexual overtones in speech and body language that border on lasciviousness (Go to #19)
   d. the employee is visually undressed, constantly touched or felt, surreptitiously kissed and/or hugged, or manipulated into being found alone (Go to #20)

17. Sexual compliance in order to keep a job or advance in it is the most common reported form of sexual harassment. You are correct.

18. Sexual availability in order to be hired is one version of sexual harassment at work. It is a less common form since most employers will defer the coercion until a later time when circumstances maximize the coercive effects. You are incorrect. (Go to #17)

19. Indirect and subtle sexual overtones are difficult to validate as sexual harassment. There may be an element of uncertainty as to whether the language or behavior is sexual harassment, discrimination, or just vulgarity and lewdness emerging in the work situation. You are incorrect. (Go to #17)

20. Women are more frequently subjected to this form of sexual harassment than men, although isolated cases of male sexual harassment are emerging in this form. People in this situation never know whether it will increase, stay the same, decrease, or stop. Most women are coerced into tolerating the pinches, feels, kisses, etc. The choice that too often exists is to tolerate the activity or to look for another job. Since it has been difficult to document the frequency of this situation, the true extent of the situation cannot be determined with accuracy. You are incorrect. (Go to #17)

PART IV REVIEW QUIZ

A. True or False

___ 1. While rape is defined as a sexual act, it is primarily an act of violence, anger, or power.

___ 2. Myths about rape have implicated the victim (usually female) in the role of being responsible for the rapist's act.

___ 3. Women frequently make false accusations of rape.

___ 4. Nonforcible rape is the most common form of rape that is reported.

___ 5. Cases of sexual intercourse between a woman and an under-age male are generally prosecuted under charges of statutory rape.

___ 6. Most researchers believe that only a small fraction of actual rapes that occur are ever reported.

___ 7. Most convicted rapists were previously convicted of rape.

___ 8. All states require the reporting of suspected incest under child abuse laws.

___ 9. Incest occurs in all walks of life and not primarily in poor, uneducated families.

___ 10. There is general agreement among men and women in top management positions on the extent of sexual harassment at work.

B. Multiple Choice--Select the Best Answer

___ 11. Coercive sex takes many different forms. All forms, however, have a key element, that being
a. sexual compliance
b. abuse of physical or social power
c. sexual harassment
d. sexual victimization

___ 12. Rape is legally defined (in most jurisdictions) by the modifying phrase
a. sexual assault
b. without mutual consent
c. penile penetration of the vagina
d. against nature

___ 13. Women who are rape victims are "blamed" for being raped based on the view that
a. women who resist can't be raped
b. women provoke men to rape them
c. women secretly want to be raped
d. all of the above

___ 14. Which of the following categories of rape is considered to be a non-forcible rape?
a. statutory rape
b. mate rape
c. date rape
d. solo rape

___ 15. Recent estimates suggest that the chances of a woman being a victim of an attempted rape during her lifetime are
a. 1 in 24
b. 1 in 12
c. 1 in 6
d. 1 in 3

___ 16. The rape victim, regardless of age, gender, or emotional state
   a. needs police protection
   b. needs careful medical attention
   c. needs psychiatric intervention
   d. needs legal advice

___ 17. A typical and dramatic sexual problem that may occur in women following a rape experience is
   a. decreased sexual desire
   b. vaginismus
   c. anorgasmia
   d. dyspareunia

___ 18. Based on studies of convicted rapists, most rapists are
   a. strangers to their victims
   b. over the age of 30 years
   c. married men
   d. well educated beyond high school

___ 19. The power-rapist usually feels
   a. a need for revenge
   b. a need to punish the victim
   c. inadequate as a person
   d. a need to make the victim suffer physical pain

___ 20. Which of the following statements about incest is a fact?
   a. Incest occurs in primarily poor, uneducated families.
   b. Incest is usually committed by a father who is a sexual degenerate.
   c. Claims of incest by a child are usually made up.
   d. None of the above.

___ 21. Most men who become involved in incestuous relationships are
   a. unconventional in other behaviors
   b. outgoing in social encounters
   c. devoted to their families
   d. all of the above

___ 22. Mother-son incest, if continued beyond the boy's age of 10 years, typically involves
   a. genital touching
   b. cunnilingus
   c. fellatio
   d. coitus

___ 23. Most researchers and clinicians agree that incest is an intensely damaging, psychological experience. It can lead to
   a. drug abuse
   b. prostitution
   c. suicide
   d. all of the above

___ 24. A survey by Redbook in 1976 that involved over 9,000 working women revealed that almost __________ percent said they had experienced some form of sexual harassment at work.
a. 90
b. 80
c. 70
d. 60

___ 25. The fundamental difference between males and females that is at the heart of sexual victimization is that
a. more men are employed in the labor force than are women
b. men are expected to be the family breadwinners
c. males are programmed for independence and aggressiveness while females are generally socialized for dependence and passivity
d. males are more sexually aggressive due to higher levels of testosterone while estrogen puts females in the position of being vulnerable to sexual abuse

PART V CLARIFYING YOUR VALUES

Sexual coercion places both men and women in "victim" roles although women are victimized more often.

The development of effective strategies to deal with the problem of coercive sex requires changing traditional gender role socialization that makes females vulnerable to sexual abuse and pushes males into the "victimizer" role. Decisions such as these are usually based upon our values and attitudes toward the use of power and influence.

The exercise that follows is designed to assist you in clarifying your choices about ways to deal with the problem of coercive sex.

COERCIVE SEX CHOICES

Instructions

Write in the feelings and behaviors you would most likely experience or engage in for each of the first eight (8) questions. In question 9, check (✓) the appropriate box to identify your choice.

1. If you were witnessing a rape of a stranger in a public place (e.g., bus depot) . . .
   a. How would you feel?

   b. What would you do?

2. If your spouse were the victim of a forcible rape . . .
   a. How would you feel?

   b. What would you do?

3. If you learned that a child in your neighborhood was being subjected to an incestuous relationship with his or her parent . . .
   a. How would you feel?

   b. What would you do?

4. If you learned that two of your children (e.g., son and daughter) were involved in brother-sister incest . . .
   a. How would you feel?

   b. What would you do?

5. If you learned that your spouse was asked to participate in sexual activity with his or her boss in order to keep a job or get a promotion . . .
   a. How would you feel?

   b. What would you do?

6. If you were applying for a position of employment that you wanted very badly and the prospective employer made it clear that hiring depended on your sexual "availability" and requested a "sample" as a sign of "good faith" . . .
   a. How would you feel?

   b. What would you do?

7. If you were constantly felt, stared at, visually and verbally "raped," and generally taken advantage of at work . . .
   a. How would you feel?

   b. What would you do?

8. If you were invited to a private showing of sexually explicit movies at a neighbor's home and realized that the films you were viewing were of young children engaged in sexual activity . . .
   a. How would you feel?

   b. What would you do?

9. If a referendum appeared on the ballot in your state to require mandatory sentences for coercive sexual behavior, how would you vote on the following? Check (√) the appropriate choice.

Coercive Sex	Sentence		
	Long Term	Short Term	None
Forcible rape			
Statutory rape			
Parent-child incest			
Sibling incest			
Sexual harassment at work			

PART VI ANSWERS TO REVIEW QUIZ

1. True. See text p. 427.
2. True. See text p. 428.
3. False. See text p. 429.
4. False. See text p. 429.
5. False. See text p. 430.
6. True. See text p. 433.
7. False. See text p. 435.
8. True. See text p. 437.
9. True. See text pp. 437-438.
10. False. See text p. 442.
11. (b) See text pp. 426-427.
12. (c) See text p. 427.
13. (d) See text p. 428.
14. (a) See text p. 430.
15. (c) See text p. 433.
16. (b) See text p. 433.
17. (b) See text p. 435.
18. (a) See text p. 435.
19. (c) See text p. 436.
20. (d) See text pp. 437-438.
21. (c) See text p. 438.
22. (d) See text p. 440.
23. (d) See text p. 440.
24. (a) See text p. 441.
25. (c) See text p. 443.

PART FIVE / CULTURAL PERSPECTIVES

18

Sexual Themes in Everyday Life

INTRODUCTION

Erotic themes in art, music, literature, media, cinema, and more recently television and advertising reflect our culture's collective attitudes toward sexuality. This chapter examines some of the ways that sexual themes permeate our lives and shape our culture's sexual identity.

PART I LEARNING OBJECTIVES

At the conclusion of this chapter, you should be able to:

1. Define pornography and obscenity.
2. Identify the historical antecedents of the U.S. obscenity laws and give examples of the materials to which they were applied.
3. Discuss the U.S. Supreme Court decisions that have both clarified and confused our current obscenity standards.
4. Summarize the findings in the 1979 Report of the Commission on Obscenity and Pornography.
5. Cite examples of the prominent literary sexual themes of several cultures throughout history.
6. Describe the recent changes in the use of erotic themes and explicit sex in the media.
7. Trace the evolution of sexual content in motion pictures and contrast the censorship practices in cinema with those in both literature and in the media.
8. Explain the reason(s) behind the more stringent censorship practices in the television industry over those in cinema.
9. List several artists and musicians who have used sexual themes in their works.
10. Discuss the opposition to sexual openness and pornography by pressure groups.

PART II IMPORTANT TERMS AND NAMES TO KNOW

A. Fill in the missing word or words.

		Key
1.	Books or pictures that depict erotic behavior with the intent of causing sexual excitement are labelled as __________. (450)	pornography
2.	Pictures or writing that is disgusting to the senses, abhorrent to morality or virtue, and/or specifically designed to incite lust or depravity are known as __________. (450)	obscenity

B. Match the name with the work.

	Name(s)	Work	Key
___	1. John Cleland (450)	a. Ulysses	Joyce
___	2. Margaret Sanger (450)	b. Lysistrata	Aristophanes
___	3. Havelock Ellis (450)	c. Cosmopolitan	Gurley-Brown
___	4. James Joyce (451, 453)	d. Leaves of Grass	Whitman
___	5. Aristophanes (452)	e. Tropic of Cancer	Miller
___	6. Petronius (452)	f. Fanny Hill	Cleland
___	7. Walt Whitman (452-453)	g. Playboy	Hefner
___	8. Henry Miller (453)	h. Studies in Psychology of Sex	Ellis
___	9. Grace Metalious (453)	i. "The Satyricon"	Petronius
___	10. Vladimir Nabokov (453)	j. Lolita	Nabokov
___	11. Hugh Hefner (455)	k. Peyton Place	Metalious
___	12. Helen Gurley Brown (455)	l. birth control	Sanger

PART III SELF-TESTING--A PROGRAMMED APPROACH

1. The handling of sexual themes by a culture gives evidence of that culture's sexual identity. In cultures that are strongly antisexual
   a. their art, literature, and dance reflect a rejecting attitude toward sex (Go to #2)
   b. their religious views are based on sexual negativism (Go to #3)
   c. there is a proliferation of obscenity laws (Go to #4)
   d. censorship is prominent and sexuality is hidden (Go to #5)

2. Art, literature, and dance most often reflect the accepting attitudes toward sex in a culture, not the rejecting ones. You are incorrect. (Go to #5)

3. There is frequently a strong correlation between religious views and sexual attitudes. The religious views today, however, are generally focused on the issue of pornography rather than sexual negativism. You are incorrect. (Go to #5)

4. The proliferation of obscenity laws that occurred during most of the 19th century has been curtailed by U.S. Supreme Court decisions over the past 25 years. You are incorrect. (Go to #5)

5. Cultures that have strong antisexual attitudes keep sexuality hidden from view and impose stringent censorship practices in order to keep it that way. You are correct. (Go to #6)

6. The major conclusion of the Commission on Obscenity and Pornography regarding the Denmark experience was that there was
   a. no significant link between adult exposure to sexual material and subsequent harmful or destructive behavior (Go to #7)
   b. a need to increase the penalties associated with pornography violations (Go to #8)
   c. insufficient sex education in the home (Go to #9)
   d. too much freedom to communicate about sexuality in the media (Go to #10)

7. Based on the study of Denmark where pornography legislation was repealed, there was no increase in sex crimes and the rates of several sex offenses declined leading the Commission to conclude that there was no significant link between adult exposure to sexual material and subsequent harmful or destructive behavior. You are correct. (Go to #11)

8. The Commission members made no mention in their report of a need to adjust penalties for pornography law breaking. In fact, they recommended a repeal of all existing pornography and obscenity laws. You are incorrect. (Go to #7)

9. While the Commission did allude to the insufficiency of sex education in the home by recommending that sex education be included in the public schools, the suggestion was based on another conclusion. You are incorrect. (Go to #7)

10. The Commission actually recommended a need for a general atmosphere of freedom to communicate about sexuality. It did not cite any form of public expression that required control or censorship. You are incorrect. (Go to #7)

11. Sexual explicitness in newspaper stories and articles <u>first</u> occurred
   a. around the turn of the 20th century (Go to #12)
   b. in the early 1950s (Go to #13)
   c. in the late 1960s (Go to #14)
   d. in the late 1970s (Go to #15)

12. Newspapers were exceedingly silent about sex in any form at the turn of the century. You are incorrect. (Go to #14)

13. Newspapers were so negative about sex in the early 1950s that many refused to carry any news stories about the Kinsey studies and some used only vague terminology about any sexual matters discussed in their columns. You are incorrect. (Go to #14)

14. Sexual words came into newsprint with the publication of <u>Human Sexual Response</u> in April of 1966. You are correct. (Go to #16)

15. By the time the 1970s came around, newspapers had stories and feature articles that discussed sex from every angle. You are incorrect. (Go to #14)

16. Critics of the upsurge of sex in advertising claim that
   a. not everyone wants to be sexy (Go to #17)
   b. it makes sexuality the prime motivation for purchase (Go to #18)
   c. too much sex detracts from the product (Go to #19)
   d. it stereotypes gender roles (Go to #20)

17. Most people in our culture equate "sexy" with attractive, desirable, and worthy of the most intimate of actions. It is a highly sought-after goal. You are incorrect. (Go to #19)

18. An ad sells a product by attracting the consumer's attention and imbedding the product's name in his or her consciousness. If sexuality gets the potential consumer's attention, it is often enough to sell the product. You are incorrect. (Go to #19)

19. Too much sex can detract from the product. Critics of the increase in sex in advertising are quick to point to this risk. You are correct.

20. Many ads still rely on stereotypical gender roles. This is beginning to change, albeit too slowly for many people. It is not the major criticism, however. You are incorrect. (Go to #19)

PART IV REVIEW QUIZ

A. True or False

___ 1. Erotic themes in everyday life tell us something about our culture's collective attitudes toward sexuality.

___ 2. The degree to which the erotic environment reflects the attitudes found in a society and the degree to which it helps shape those attitudes is not always apparent.

___ 3. The first conviction for selling obscene literature in the U.S. occurred in the Commonwealth of Massachusetts. The book was Ulysses.

___ 4. Obscenity in the 1600s meant blasphemy and had nothing to do with sexual content or material.

___ 5. Many books that are now recognized as literary classics were prohibited or banned by obscenity laws during the first part of the 20th century.

___ 6. In 1973, the U.S. Supreme Court ruled that local community standards could be used to obtain obscenity convictions.

___ 7. Most newspaper editorials about the Kinsey reports reflected approval of both the subject of human sexual behavior and the findings.

___ 8. In the late 1970s there were several write-in campaigns to large advertisers insisting on the ban of sexually-oriented programming.

___ 9. The heyday of erotic art was during the Renaissance.

___ 10. The real sexual revolutionaries in the rock'n roll music world were the Beatles.

B. Multiple Choice--Select the Best Answer

___ 11. According to U.S. law
a. pornography and obscenity are illegal
b. pornography is legal, obscenity is illegal
c. pornography is illegal, obscenity is legal
d. pornography and obscenity are both legal

___ 12. During the 1600s U.S. obscenity laws were based on the notion that
a. public display of sexual material was obscene
b. indecent books and pictures were pornographic
c. obscenity was an offense against religion
d. sexual materials corrupted public morals

___ 13. During most of the 19th century, state and federal obscenity laws and statutes were
a. seldom enforced
b. strictly enforced
c. repealed
d. rewritten to include harsher penalties

____ 14. The federal mail act to prohibit the mailing of obscene literature and allow the post office to confiscate it was championed by
a. Margaret Sanger
b. Havelock Ellis
c. Charles Rembar
d. Anthony Comstock

____ 15. The definition of obscenity that was handed down by the U.S. Supreme Court in 1966 and still used today to determine obscenity cases is that the material in question
a. must appeal to a prurient interest in sex
b. must offend contemporary community standards
c. is utterly without redeeming social value
d. all of the above

____ 16. One of the problems that this judicial decision of the Supreme Court produced was
a. uncertainty about what constitutes a community
b. the basis for judging social value
c. uncertainty about what constitutes the "average person"
d. all of the above

____ 17. The President's Commission on Obscenity and Pornography (1970) recommended
a. repeal of all existing pornography and obscenity laws
b. the exclusion of sex education from the public schools
c. greater controls on the media
d. all of the above

____ 18. One of the most repressive times in history regarding sexual material ironically produced an underground world of erotic literature. This period was known as the
a. Renaissance
b. Victorian Era
c. Roaring Twenties
d. Nuclear Age

____ 19. Although James Joyce's classic book, _Ulysses_, became available in the U.S. following the decision of Judge Woolsey, two other sexually explicit novels were banned until the late 1950s. These were
a. _Peyton Place_ and _Lolita_
b. _Lady Chatterley's Lover_ and _Tropic of Cancer_
c. _My Secret Life_ and _Leaves of Grass_
d. all of the above

____ 20. Newspapers were reluctant to publish stories and feature articles discussing sex until the publication of
a. the _Redbook_ Study
b. the _Playboy_ Survey
c. _The Hite Report_
d. none of the above

___ 21. The leader in women's magazines for the inclusion of sexual themes was
   a. Cosmopolitan
   b. Redbook
   c. McCalls
   d. Ms.

___ 22. The acceptability of sex on the screen today is determined by
   a. censorship boards
   b. box office success
   c. the Motion Picture Association of America
   d. the Adult Film Association of America

___ 23. Sex in cinema during the later 1970s and early 1980s
   a. centered on explicit sexual acts
   b. was noticeably absent from films
   c. was woven into the stories by focusing more on the person rather than the sexual acts
   d. exploited the seamy side of brutality in sex

___ 24. Sex on television was even more heavily censored than the movie industry had been. The frankness of one TV show in particular opened the gates for sexual themes on television. The show was titled
   a. Mary Hartman, Mary Hartman
   b. All the Days in Your Lives
   c. All in the Family
   d. Soap

___ 25. The symbolism of sex in rock 'n roll has been identified with the gyrations of
   a. Elvis Presley
   b. Chuck Berry
   c. The Beatles
   d. Mick Jagger

PART V CLARIFYING YOUR VALUES

We have seen that our current cultural attitudes and uncertainties about sex are mirrored in the sexual themes that permeate our lives. The degree to which our erotic environment shapes our attitudes is not always apparent.

The exercise that follows is intended to help you conceptualize this more clearly.

INFLUENCE OF EROTICA

1. Identify your feelings about the degree to which your erotic environment affected your sexual attitudes by placing a check (√) in the appropriate space.

	Attitudinal Influences					
	Childhood		Adolescence		Adulthood	
Erotic Environment	Major	Minor	Major	Minor	Major	Minor
1. Obscenity						
2. Pornography						
3. Erotic books						
4. Erotic magazines						
5. Erotic newspapers						
6. Erotic art						
7. Erotic music						
8. Erotic movies						
9. Erotic TV						
10. Other?						

2. Go back over the checkmarks. List the sources of sexual themes for each of the major influences that you have checked.

Example: Erotic Books
Childhood - Steffie Can't Come Out to Play
Adolescence -
Adulthood - Couples

Erotic Magazines
Childhood -
Adolescence - Playboy (my father's copy)
Adulthood - Hustler

3. In what ways have these affected your sexual attitudes?

PART VI ANSWERS TO REVIEW QUIZ

1. True. See text p. 449.
2. True. See text p. 450.
3. False. See text p. 450.
4. True. See text p. 450.
5. True. See text p. 450.
6. True. See text p. 451.
7. False. See text p. 454.
8. True. See text p. 458.
9. False. See text p. 462.
10. False. See text p. 463.
11. (b) See text p. 450.
12. (c) See text p. 450.
13. (a) See text p. 450.
14. (d) See text p. 450.
15. (d) See text p. 451.
16. (d) See text p. 451.
17. (a) See text pp. 451-452.
18. (b) See text p. 452.
19. (b) See text p. 453.
20. (d) See text p. 455.
21. (a) See text p. 455.
22. (b) See text p. 456.
23. (c) See text p. 456.
24. (c) See text p. 457.
25. (a) See text pp. 462-463.

19

Religious and Ethical Perspectives on Sexuality

INTRODUCTION

All religions have dealt with sexuality in some manner. While they have changed to some extent over the course of time, religious views still have an effect upon our personal and cultural values. This chapter examines the two major ways we approach questions of values in order to make sexual choices: through religious beliefs and ethical analysis. It includes discussions of three sexual issues that are a source of ethical and religious controversy: (1) abortion, (2) homosexuality, and (3) contraception.

PART I LEARNING OBJECTIVES

At the conclusion of this chapter, you should be able to:

1. Describe the similarities and differences in the ways particular religions have handled sexual issues.
2. Contrast ethical questions about sex with those based on personal taste and preference.
3. Identify the four moral views by which educated people judge the moral appropriateness of a sexual act.
4. Discuss the historical background and attitudes about abortion and state the three primary positions that people take on abortion.
5. Explain the position(s) most religions take in regard to homosexuality.
6. Compare and contrast the views regarding contraception methods held by different religious groups.
7. List the major ethical questions concerning contraception.
8. Briefly summarize the religious teachings about sexuality included in Islam, Hinduism, and Buddhism.

PART II IMPORTANT TERMS AND NAMES TO KNOW

Fill in the missing word, words, or names.

1. __________ __________ viewed every sexual act, even marital coitus, as sinful. (469) — St. Augustine
2. __________ __________ led a split from the Catholic Church due in part to the fact that his sexual attitudes were at variance with the Church's, especially over the issue of celibacy. (472) — Martin Luther
3. The conservative group within Protestantism whose views on sexuality are almost indistinguishable from those of Catholicism are known as __________. (473) — fundamentalists
4. __________ __________ are a religious group who follow the Bible literally in finding rules for sexual behavior. (473) — Jehovah's Witnesses
5. __________ define the integrity of the relationship between the people as the measure for sexual morality. (473-474) — Quakers
6. Those people who take the position that abortion should be banned under all circumstances are known as the pro __________ group. (475-476) — life
7. Those people who take the position that abortion should be available to all pregnant women at their request are known as the pro __________ group. (476) — choice
8. __________, a religion born in the Middle East, takes a very positive view of most forms of sexuality including polygamy. (471) — Islam

9. __________, the founder of Islam, recorded his views on sexuality in the Koran. (471) — Muhammed

10. __________, the oldest religion in India, is a collection of many different approaches to life, including a number of different sexual philosophies. (471) — Hinduism

11. A book written by a Hindu priest that provides detailed discussions and illustrations of sexual techniques and coital positions is the __________ __________. (471) — Kama Sutra

12. __________, founded in India, is a religion that stresses celibacy as a form of mental and moral self-purification. (471) — Buddhism

PART III SELF-TESTING--A PROGRAMMED APPROACH

1. The basic attitude that sexuality is a positive force, a gift of God, lends itself to the view that the joy of sexual activity is good in and of itself, apart from procreative potential. Which of the following religions profess this attitude?
   a. Judaism (Go to #2)
   b. Catholicism (Go to #3)
   c. Protestantism (Go to #4)
   d. Hinduism (Go to #5)

2. Jewish views on sexuality are based on the notion that since God created man and woman in his own image, it would be irreverent to regard the sex organs or their functions as obscene. You are correct. (Go to #6)

3. Catholic views on sexuality hold that sexual activity in marriage is good as long as it has the potential for reproduction. You are incorrect. (Go to #2)

4. Protestant views on sexuality hold that sexual activity in marriage is good although there is such a diversity of attitudes regarding other sexual behaviors that it is difficult to label a Protestant perspective. You are incorrect. (Go to #2)

5. Hinduism holds that approaches to life differ, therefore a variety of sexual philosophies emerge. The path of Karma is closest to the basic attitude described above; however, it is only one of several approaches. You are incorrect. (Go to #2)

6. Overall, there seems to be a feeling by many American clergy that cut-and-dried pronouncements on the morality of sexual behavior should be avoided. Instead they recommend
   a. establishing cultural standards (Go to #7)
   b. updating sexual doctrines (Go to #8)
   c. providing flexible and inventive counseling (Go to #9)
   d. developing dialogue about sex (Go to #10)

7. Cultural standards are a form of cut-and-dried pronouncement. You are incorrect. (Go to #10)

8. Updating sexual doctrines is a form of generalizing and does not consider the relative merits of each individual situation. You are incorrect. (Go to #10)

9. Flexible and inventive counseling can be an excellent approach to the pastoral function. It is limited, however, to that function and does not reflect the breadth of the moral issues involved in sexual behavior. You are incorrect. (Go to #10)

10. Most American clergy are in favor of a developing dialogue about sex. You are correct. (Go to #11)

11. Sexual decisions are made on a variety of considerations. Some are ethically "value free"; others are ethical questions. Those that are "value-loaded" require
    a. faith (Go to #12)
    b. a process of rational thought (Go to #13)
    c. cognitive dissonance (Go to #14)
    d. personal taste and preference (Go to #15)

12. Faith is used to make moral decisions based solely on religion. You are incorrect. (Go to #13)

13. A process of rational thought is required for ethical decision making since difficult ethical problems are those that do not present black and white choices. You are correct. (Go to #16)

14. Cognitive dissonance is used to invalidate beliefs based on facts and information. These are not "value-laden" ethical issues; rather, they are knowledge or epistemological issues. You are incorrect. (Go to #13)

15. Personal taste and preference are used to reach decisions that are ethically "value-free"; that is, they are not a matter of "right" and "wrong" in a moral sense. You are incorrect. (Go to #13)

16. College-educated people tend to judge the moral appropriateness of a sexual act on which of the following standards?
    a. whether the sex act was satisfying for both partners (Go to #17)
    b. whether the participants had a long-term relationship (Go to #18)
    c. whether there was a commitment for mutual growth (Go to #19)
    d. whether the two people really loved each other (Go to #20)

17. College-educated people do not equate sexual satisfaction with morality or ethics. You are incorrect. (Go to #20)

18. A long-term relationship would only be important to college-educated people if it enhanced the interpersonal relationship. You are incorrect. (Go to #20)

19. Commitment would be an ethical issue if personal growth and development could be enhanced by it. Most college-educated people judge the morality issue more on the basis of all the facts of a given situation rather than on some absolute rule such as commitment. You are incorrect. (Go to #20)

20. The primary standard used by college-educated people to judge the appropriateness of a sexual act is whether the two people really loved each other. You are correct.

PART IV REVIEW QUIZ

A. True or False

___ 1. Jewish tradition valued marriage as existing only for the purpose of having children.

___ 2. Jewish law urges that all people marry including those who are infertile or elderly.

___ 3. Christianity was often outspoken and positive about human sexuality as a gift from God.

___ 4. St. Augustine viewed every sexual act--even marital intercourse--as sinful.

___ 5. The Catholic church does not permit divorce except under special circumstances.

___ 6. Martin Luther's most conspicuous change in sexual attitude was his rejection of the Church's ban on divorce.

___ 7. There is little diversity of opinion about sexual matters among the Protestant denominations.

___ 8. Many people who consider themselves religious find that their sexual decisions often are in conflict with the teaching of their religion.

___ 9. Kinsey concluded that formal religious affiliations influenced people's views of sexual morality more than their educational level.

___ 10. Every known religion has teachings that relate to sexual ethics and they tend to all agree on two issues: adultery and homosexuality.

B. Multiple Choice--Select the Best Answer

___ 11. Jewish views on sexuality stem from
a. Old Testament and the Talmud
b. Code of Hammurabi and Mosiac Law
c. Ten Commandments and Prophecies
d. the Torah and Covenants

___ 12. Judaism condemns certain forms of sexual behavior including
a. oral sex
b. prostitution
c. lesbianism
d. celibacy

___ 13. The early disciples of Jesus seem to have been strongly influenced by which of the following views about physical-spiritual love?
a. Jewish
b. Greek
c. Roman
d. Arabic

___ 14. The sexuality position of the Catholic Church is based on the
a. Old Testament and the Epistles
b. New Testament and Vatican Councils
c. Old and New Testaments and teachings of the Popes
d. all of the above

___ 15. The 1981 meeting of U.S. and Canadian Catholic bishops pointed out that the primary role of sexual union is
a. to produce children
b. to enable each person to reach fulfillment
c. to propagate the faith
d. to validate marriage

___ 16. Martin Luther encouraged priests and nuns to marry because
a. they possessed no special divine authority
b. there was no religious meaning to the effort to be especially holy
c. he saw sex as a natural part of human life
d. all of the above

___ 17. The Protestant Reformation continued traditional Christian ideals in sexual matters by viewing which of the following as sinful?
a. masturbation
b. abortion
c. contraception
d. all of the above

___ 18. Fundamentalists are grouped into which of the following classifications of Protestant perspectives?
a. conservative
b. moderate
c. liberal
d. evangelical

___ 19. Moderate Protestants believe that divorce is
   a. sinful
   b. not a religious matter
   c. often the lesser evil to a tormented marriage
   d. inconsistent with Christian ethics

___ 20. Quakers measure sexual morality as
   a. the greatest good for the greatest number
   b. individual choice unless it harms another person
   c. the integrity of the relationship between the people involved
   d. all of the above

___ 21. Which of the following questions about sexual decisions is ethically "value-free"?
   a. Am I being honest?
   b. Am I doing the right thing?
   c. Is there a chance I'll hurt my partner?
   d. Is this the right time and place?

___ 22. Which of the following is <u>not</u> a primary position taken by people on the abortion issue?
   a. Abortions should be banned under all circumstances.
   b. A physician may not refuse to perform an abortion.
   c. Abortions should be restricted to certain situations.
   d. Abortion should be available to all pregnant women at their request.

___ 23. Which of the following propositions does the "Pro-Life" movement espouse?
   a. Enforced maternities should not take place.
   b. Human life begins at the moment of conception.
   c. Male domination is responsible for stringent abortion laws.
   d. Female freedom is dependent on a woman's control of her procreative life.

___ 24. Religious attitudes toward homosexuality have shifted to a point where all religions agree that
   a. homosexuality is an illness
   b. homosexuality is a sin
   c. pastoral care should be available to homosexual persons
   d. homosexual expression between consenting adults is not immoral

___ 25. To Western observers, the one religion that appears to be severely biased against women is
   a. Hinduism
   b. Buddhism
   c. Islam
   d. all of the above

PART V CLARIFYING YOUR VALUES

This chapter suggested that there was no single set of rules or ethical standards that suit all people in all societies all of the time. In fact, many people who consider themselves to be religious find that they often make sexual decisions that conflict with the teachings of their religion. While this has occurred for centuries, it may be more pronounced today in light of the rapidly changing cultural attitudes about sexuality.

The exercise that follows is intended to clarify some of the ethical and religious ideas that may have had an influence on your sexual attitudes. Hopefully, it will assist you in sorting out your values in the tug-of-war that often exists between those traditional teachings and contemporary cultural attitudes.

Read the statements in the left-hand column. Indicate your agreement-disagreement with each statement and identify whether this attitude is consistent or inconsistent with the views espoused by your religion or ethical analysis. Place a check (√) in the appropriate box.

CLARIFYING RELIGIOUS AND ETHICAL PERSPECTIVES

Statements	Attitude: Agree	Attitude: Disagree	Religious View/Ethics: Consistent	Religious View/Ethics: Inconsistent
1. Sex and love are independent; sex should be enjoyed for its own sake.				
2. Premarital coitus is wrong; couples should wait until marriage.				
3. There is nothing wrong with being gay; homosexual acts are not immoral.				
4. Extramarital sex adds a dimension to marriage; there is nothing wrong with it.				
5. Anyone who wants to prevent pregnancy should have access to contraception; it doesn't matter whether a person is married or not or young or old.				
6. Any woman should have the right to have an abortion; it is her decision, no one else's.				
7. The best source of sex education for children is the church or synagogue; schools have no business including it in the curriculum.				
8. Prostitution is wrong; prostitutes should be subject to harsh fines and sentences.				
9. Women should feel free to initiate sexual activity; they should take an active role in love-making.				
10. Sexuality is a positive force; a gift of God, meant to be enjoyed.				
11. Masturbation is a moral disorder; it is a sinful act.				
12. Chastity is virtuous; it attains a higher spiritual good.				
13. Divorce should be more difficult to obtain; marriage should be a life-long commitment.				
14. Any private sexual activity between consenting adults is moral; it is a matter of conscience.				

Are any of your attitudes in conflict with the views of your religious faith or ethical principles?

If they are, why do you think these conflicts exist?

PART VI ANSWERS TO REVIEW QUIZ

1. False. See text p. 468.
2. True. See text p. 468.
3. False. See text p. 469.
4. True. See text p. 469.
5. True. See text p. 472.
6. False. See text p. 472.
7. False. See text p. 473.
8. True. See text p. 474.
9. False. See text p. 475.
10. False. See text p. 471.
11. (a) See text p. 468.
12. (d) See text p. 468.
13. (b) See text p. 469.
14. (c) See text p. 469.
15. (b) See text p. 472.
16. (a) See text pp. 472-473.
17. (a) See text p. 473.
18. (a) See text p. 473.
19. (c) See text p. 473.
20. (c) See text pp. 473-474.
21. (d) See text p. 474.
22. (b) See text pp. 475-476.
23. (b) See text p. 476.
24. (c) See text p. 480.
25. (c) See text p. 471.

20
Sexuality in Cross-Cultural Perspective

INTRODUCTION

This final chapter brings our study of human sexuality full circle. Cross-cultural studies provide a particularly effective vehicle for a concluding examination of sex because the sexual impulse is universal among the human species. This approach allows us to objectively reevaluate our previously unquestioned ideas and challenge our culture-bound assumptions. The chapter draws upon the cross-cultural study method of anthropology to expose the influence that cultures have on the sexual attitudes and behaviors of their people. It includes the cross-cultural study of sexual attraction, early sexual activity, solitary sexual activity, premarital heterosexuality, sex and marriage, homosexuality, paraphilias, and ritualized sex.

PART I LEARNING OBJECTIVES

At the conclusion of this chapter, you should be able to:

1. Explain why sex is particularly well-suited for cross-cultural studies.
2. Describe the physical characteristics of sexually attractive persons in all cultures, the sexual attractiveness of other physical attributes that depend on the values of the culture, and the behavioral patterns of sexually attractive persons in most cultures.
3. Compare and contrast the culturally approved and condemned forms of sexuality among cultures during childhood and puberty.
4. Identify the premarital heterosexual behaviors practiced in our European-American culture and shared by other cultures.
5. Discuss the relationship between sex and marriage in those cultures in which the union of sexual partners is legitimized and list the benefits of marriage and the societal rules and regulations for marriage.
6. Compare the types of marriages and the attitudes toward them by various cultures.

7. Discuss the way in which extramarital activity is handled by various societies.
8. Contrast the varying styles of handling male and female homosexuality in different societies.
9. Explain why paraphilias are almost unheard of in preindustrial societies.
10. Discuss the significance of ceremonial, religious, and ritualized forms of sex.

PART II IMPORTANT TERMS TO KNOW

Fill in the missing word or words.

1.	__________ were male demons believed during the Middle Ages to copulate with sleeping women, thus entering their bodies and influencing their behavior. (489)	incubi
2.	__________ were female demons believed during the Middle Ages to copulate with sleeping men, thus entering their bodies and influencing their behavior. (489)	succubi
3.	The tendency to marry one's relatives or within one's group is called __________. (492)	endogamy
4.	The tendency to marry outside one's relatives or group is called __________. (492)	exogamy
5.	Specifying exactly whom one should marry is known as __________ __________. (492)	preferential marriage
6.	A brief time when ordinary sexual restraints become inoperative because of some ceremony, ritual, or celebration is called __________ __________. (498)	ceremonial license

PART III SELF-TESTING--A PROGRAMMED APPROACH

1. Sex is particularly suited for cross-cultural studies because
   a. sex is significantly influenced by environmental factors (Go to #2)
   b. the sexual impulse is shared by virtually all human beings (Go to #3)
   c. human sexual capacities are learned or conditioned (Go to #4)
   d. cross-cultural studies reinforce our culture-bound ideas (Go to #5)

2. Sex is influenced little by environmental factors except for disease and malnutrition. Factors such as temperature, altitude, water, weather, and soil affect our living conditions but not our sexual behaviors. You are incorrect. (Go to #3)

3. The sexual drive is shared by virtually all human beings and exists in most of humankind for the duration of their lives. You are correct. (Go to #6)

4. Human sexual capacities are limited by genetics, biology, and evolution. These limits are not set by learning and conditioning, although learning and conditioning can cause enormous differences in sexual behaviors and capacities. You are incorrect. (Go to #3)

5. Cross-cultural studies can dissolve culture-bound ideas and help people see and appreciate the realities and possibilities in their own lives. You are incorrect. (Go to #3)

6. Physical sexual attractiveness is basically determined by
   a. body symmetry (Go to #7)
   b. health and the absence of disease or infirmity (Go to #8)
   c. skeletal structure (Go to #9)
   d. the values placed on physical attributes by the particular culture (Go to #10)

7. Although body symmetry is considered to be a factor in determining physical attractiveness in some cultures, many cultures value over- or undersized body parts such as buttocks or breasts. Body symmetry is not the most basic determinant of physical attractiveness. You are incorrect. (Go to #10)

8. Reasonable health is a fairly common criterion for physical attractiveness, although overly robust individuals can be unattractive to many people (e.g., body builders) while pale, frail, and delicate females (e.g., Camille) are sexually attractive in many cultures. Health is not the basic determinant of physical attractiveness in most cultures. You are incorrect. (Go to #10)

9. Skeletal structure is important for physical attractiveness only to the degree that all of the body parts are in place, hence people who have missing limbs or extra appendages (e.g., amputees, thalidomide deformities, extra fingers, etc.) are less physically attractive. But skeletal structure is not the basic determinant of physical attractiveness. You are incorrect. (Go to #10)

10. While all of the other factors (i.e., body symmetry, health, skeletal structure) play a role in determining physical attractiveness, the basic determinant of what constitutes physical attractiveness remains the values placed on physical attributes by the particular culture (e.g., thin women in the U.S. vs. fat women in certain African cultures). You are correct. (Go to #11)

11. Most cultures have ceremonies and rituals to mark or recognize the transition point between childhood and adulthood called puberty. The most striking difference between Western societies and the others is the Western practice of
  a. involving the adolescent boy or girl in symbolic or educative sexual acts (Go to #12)
  b. exposing the adolescent boy or girl to physical discomfort or pain (e.g., genital operations) (Go to #13)
  c. allowing certain changes in dress and cosmetics and by regarding all subsequent male-female relationships as being potentially sexual (Go to #14)
  d. encouraging homosexual acts as a way of preparing the adolescent for sexual maturity (Go to #15)

12. Sexual acts are used more typically in the South Seas such as on the Polynesian Island of Mangaia. They are not typical for Western societies even though many adolescent males sometimes fabricate stories to the contrary. You are incorrect. (Go to #14)

13. Puberty rites often include genital operations such as circumcision or branding body parts as a mark of puberty. They involve pain and discomfort especially when a body part is drastically assaulted or disfigured. These practices are more common in non-Western cultures. You are incorrect. (Go to #14)

14. Western society does not have puberty ceremonies (bar or bas mitzvah's, confirmations, etc., notwithstanding) per se, but does commemorate puberty by altering certain dress and cosmetic standards and viewing male-female interactions as potentially sexual. You are correct. (Go to #16)

15. Male puberty rites in a New Guinea tribe include homosexual activity. It is a rare ritual and one not typical of Western societies. You are incorrect. (Go to #14)

16. Nearly all people in the world agree that the incest taboo is genetically and socially determined. This agreement destroys the myth that people developed the incest taboo because
  a. it confused kinship and inheritance laws (Go to #17)
  b. they recognized the detrimental effects of inbreeding (Go to #18)
  c. it would cause role conflicts (Go to #19)
  d. it made life unworkably complicated (Go to #20)

17. Kinship and inheritance confusion were a reality, not a myth. You are incorrect. (Go to #18)

18. Recognition of the detrimental effects of inbreeding is a myth. Social issues were involved. You are correct.

19. Role conflicts were an important social factor in the incest taboo. It was not part of the myth. You are incorrect. (Go to #18)

20. The simplest reason why virtually all people have some sort of incest taboo is that incest would make life unworkably complicated. It is definitely not a myth. You are incorrect. (Go to #18)

PART IV REVIEW QUIZ

A. True or False

___ 1. The sexual attractiveness of nudity is culturally determined.

___ 2. Male sexual attractiveness seems enhanced in all societies by behavior which indicates the male is socially successful.

___ 3. In the U.S. and Western Europe, female attractiveness is enhanced by the suggestion of sexual unavailability.

___ 4. Socially approved sexual contact between children and adults is fairly common in human history.

___ 5. Masturbation is a common practice in sexually permissive societies.

___ 6. All societies have rules as to whom one can or cannot marry.

___ 7. All societies tend to allow or forgive extramarital activity by males and to be more harsh toward such behavior by females.

___ 8. Most societies allow postmarital persons far less sexual freedom than that permitted to the never-married or married.

___ 9. Predominant homosexuality as a lifetime pattern is very rare in preindustrial societies.

___ 10. Paraphilias are more commonly found in preindustrial societies than in Western industrial ones.

B. Multiple Choice--Select the Best Answer

___ 11. The processes of learning and conditioning operate within the limits set by
a. evolution
b. biology
c. genetics
d. all of the above

___ 12. It appears that the differences in sexual behavior and capacities
a. are less than differences in other universal behaviors and capacities
b. are about the same as differences in other universal behaviors and capacities
c. are greater than the differences in other universal behaviors and capacities
d. cannot be ascertained from the limited anthropological studies on human sexuality

___ 13. What is considered sexually stimulating in most societies is
a. always in terms of the male's response to female exposure
b. always in terms of the female's response to male exposure
c. determined by societal leaders (male or female)
d. depends on whether they are industrial or preindustrial societies

___ 14. Novelty of new sexual partners is perceived as more sexually stimulating in
a. industrial societies
b. preindustrial societies
c. a few primitive cultures
d. most cultures

___ 15. Sexual attractiveness is diminished by
a. social success
b. domestic skills
c. close rearing
d. social availability

___ 16. Socially approved sexual contact between children and adults is permitted in only a few societies and generally only in the form of
a. pedophilia
b. child marriage
c. incest
d. soothing fretful infants by masturbating them

___ 17. Most societies mark the occasion of puberty by
a. a ceremony at the time of onset of menses
b. a ceremony when first orgasm is reached
c. having one or a few ceremonies per year to accommodate those who reached puberty during that time
d. individualized rituals involving physical discomfort and pain

___ 18. If one adds the societies which publicly deplore premarital coitus but secretly condone it to those societies which permit it between certain persons and under certain conditions, the percentage of "permissive" societies would be about
a. 25%
b. 50%
c. 75%
d. 100%

___ 19. The great value that some societies attach to female virginity is the result of
a. viewing females as property
b. wanting one's children to be one's own
c. avoiding an experienced female who would not only have sexual expectations, but who would be in a position to make comparisons
d. all of the above

___ 20. A benefit of marriage is that it
a. enables two people to live as cheaply as one
b. legitimizes sexual relationships
c. establishes new kinships
d. provides emotional security for both partners

___ 21. In societies that have few or no restrictions on the frequency of coitus, coitus averages about __________ per week during middle age.
a. once
b. twice
c. three times
d. four times

___ 22. While most societies seemingly forbid and punish extramarital sex, on closer inspection one finds that
a. it is permitted in certain clearly defined circumstances
b. it seldom leads to divorce
c. it improves most marriages
d. all of the above

___ 23. The reason that we know very little about female homosexuality is that
a. most anthropologists have been male
b. most anthropologists were reticent about studying sex
c. most anthropologists are very naive about female sexuality
d. all of the above

___ 24. Anthropology has shown that homosexuality
a. is more commonly a predominant lifelong pattern in preindustrial societies
b. is frequently divided for males into the penetrator and the penetrated
c. and heterosexuality are mutually exclusive
d. is the product of conditioning by previous behavior

___ 25. Paraphilias are believed to be associated with
a. dependence on and use of symbolism
b. sexual restraints in early childhood
c. painful rituals
d. all of the above

PART V CLARIFYING YOUR VALUES

Most people will agree that no sexual act bears an inherent social or psychological value for good or evil: the value and meaning of any act are determined by the social context in which it occurs. The exercise that follows is intended to help you clarify your values about certain sexual acts and contrast them against the cultural experiment that you are a part of as a college student in the United States of America.

CONTRASTING CULTURAL AND PERSONAL VALUES

Instructions

Place a check (√) under the appropriate response indicating the prevailing cultural value regarding certain sexual acts and your own personal value about the "rightness" or "wrongness" of the sexual act.

Sexual Act	Cultural Value		Personal Value	
	Right	Wrong	Right	Wrong
1. Public nudity				
2. Masturbation (in private)				
3. Childhood sex play				
4. Premarital coitus				
5. Endogamy				
6. Exogamy				
7. Incest				
8. Extramarital coitus				
9. Postmarital coitus				
10. Male homosexuality				
11. Female homosexuality				
12. Paraphilias				
13. Ritualized sex				
14. Other(s)?				

PART VI ANSWERS TO REVIEW QUIZ

1. True. See text p. 485.
2. True. See text p. 487.
3. False. See text p. 487.
4. False. See text p. 487.
5. False. See text p. 489.
6. True. See text p. 490.
7. True. See text p. 494.
8. False. See text p. 495.
9. True. See text p. 497.
10. False. See text p. 497.
11. (d) See text p. 485.
12. (c) See text p. 485.
13. (a) See text p. 486.
14. (d) See text pp. 486-487.
15. (c) See text p. 487.
16. (b) See text p. 487.
17. (c) See text p. 488.
18. (c) See text p. 490.
19. (d) See text p. 490.
20. (c) See text p. 492.
21. (b) See text p. 494.
22. (a) See text p. 495.
23. (d) See text p. 496.
24. (b) See text p. 497.
25. (a) See text pp. 497-498.

SKAT
SEXUAL KNOWLEDGE AND ATTITUDE TEST
POSTTEST

This test is divided into two sections: Part One contains 40 questions on sexual knowledge; Part Two contains 20 statements about your sexual attitudes.

Instructions for responding to each section are found at the beginning of each section.

Correct answers for the knowledge section (Part One) and scoring directions for the attitude section (Part Two) are found at the end of Part Two of this Posttest.

It should take you about 30 minutes to complete the SKAT Posttest.

Instructions for comparing the scores and changes which have occurred are found at the end of this Posttest.

Do not complete this Posttest until you have finished the material in the Study Guide (Chapters 1 - 20).

This test is based on material covered in the textbook and in classroom learning activities. Therefore, your participation in class sessions, your reading of the textbook, and completion of the exercises in this Study Guide, have probably changed both your knowledge and attitudes about human sexuality. By comparing your scores on this Posttest with those on the Pretest, you can measure the extent of these changes.

PART ONE - KNOWLEDGE

True or False (Circle your answer)

T F 1. Our sexual attitudes and beliefs are largely influenced by psychosocial factors.

T F 2. The uterus is part of the internal female sex organs.

T F 3. Vasocongestion and increased neuromuscular tension are the two basic physiologic responses during human sexual response.

T F 4. The first stage of labor begins with effacement and dilatation.

T F 5. The most serious risk to women using birth control pills is the high probability of developing malignancies.

T F 6. A chemical substance, H-Y antigen, which is controlled by the Y chromosome, is necessary to start testes development in the male embryo.

T F 7. There is a considerable amount of reliable data about sexual behavior during childhood.

T F 8. Mothers talk more to their male infants than to their female infants.

T F 9. Caring and respect for the other person is a central feature of sexual passion.

T F 10. People who insist on keeping sexual fantasies private are generally immature and emotionally unready for an intimate sexual relationship.

T F 11. Sexual self-stimulation which does not lead to orgasm is not considered to be masturbation.

T F 12. The frequency of marital intercourse declines with the length of marriage.

T F 13. Gay men are more likely than lesbians to have difficulty accepting their homosexuality.

T F 14. Paraphilias are more common in women than in men.

T F 15. It is not always possible to precisely identify the cause of a specific sexual dysfunction in a given person.

T F 16. Syphilis is the oldest and most common form of STD.

T F 17. Women frequently make false accusations of rape.

T F 18. Erotic themes in everyday life gives us clues to our culture's collective attitudes toward sexuality.

T F 19. Many American clergy feel that cut-and-dried pronouncements on the morality of sexual behavior should be avoided.

T F 20. Most cultures hold that the incest taboo is genetically and socially determined.

Multiple Choice (Circle your answer)

21. The most controversial type of sex research is
    a. observational study
    b. interview survey
    c. case study
    d. questionnaire survey

22. Sperm cells are produced in the
    a. seminiferous tubules
    b. epididymis
    c. vas deferens
    d. seminal vesicles

23. The major difference between male and female sexual response immediately following orgasm is the fact that
    a. all women experience multiple orgasm
    b. men have a refractory period, women do not
    c. women need constant physical stimulation to keep aroused
    d. women do not experience orgasm during sleep

24. During normal delivery, the baby's position is in the
    a. breech presentation
    b. cephalic presentation
    c. transverse presentation
    d. longitudinal presentation

25. The birth control technique that depends on changes in the cervical mucus is the
    a. calendar method
    b. temperature method
    c. ovulation method
    d. enzyme method

26. Sexual differentiation starts from the moment of conception and is largely controlled by
    a. chromosomes
    b. hormones
    c. a combination of genetic and hormonal mechanisms
    d. the embryonic duct system

27. Children in our society usually begin asking questions about how babies are made and how birth occurs by the time they are
    a. able to speak
    b. toilet trained
    c. four years old
    d. in school

28. Core gender identity is well established by the time a child reaches
    a. the end of the first year of life
    b. the age of 3 years old
    c. school age
    d. puberty

29. In any type of love, the one element that is essential is
    a. passion for the person
    b. friendship with the person
    c. dependency on the person
    d. caring about the person

30. The primary fascination with a preferential sexual fantasy lies in its
    a. recurring nature
    b. pleasing effect
    c. familiar theme
    d. sexual arousal

31. Masturbation usually
    a. begins in childhood
    b. begins in adolescence
    c. is terminated after marriage
    d. continues in the older adult who is emotionally unstable

32. The percentage of women who are orgasmic during premarital coitus has been
    a. increasing
    b. decreasing
    c. unchanged
    d. not researched adequately

33. Homosexuality is caused by
    a. biological factors
    b. psychological factors
    c. family patterns
    d. no known specific causes

34. A paraphilia which often leads to theft of another person's personal property is
    a. fetishism
    b. transvestism
    c. frotteurism
    d. klismaphilia

35. Females who are affected by vaginismus are generally
    a. in their adolescence
    b. in their early 20s
    c. past the age of 35
    d. of any age

36. Most spinal cord injured men
    a. lose the ability to have normal erections
    b. lose the ability to ejaculate
    c. become infertile
    d. all of the above

37. A typical and dramatic sexual problem that may occur in women following a rape experience is
    a. decreased sexual desire
    b. vaginismus
    c. anorgasmia
    d. dyspareunia

38. The President's Commission on Obscenity and Pornography (1970) recommended
    a. repeal of all existing pornography and obscenity laws
    b. the exclusion of sex education from the public schools
    c. greater controls upon the media
    d. all of the above

39. Jewish views on sexuality stem from the
    a. Old Testament and the Talmud
    b. Code of Hammurabi and Mosiac Law
    c. Ten Commandments and Prophecies
    d. Torah and Covenants

40. In most cultures, sexual attractiveness is diminished by
    a. social success
    b. domestic skills
    c. close rearing
    d. social availability

PART TWO - ATTITUDE

Respond to each statement in the following ways:

SA - Circle if you Strongly Agree with the statement.
A - Circle if you Moderately Agree with the statement.
N - Circle if you have no opinion.
D - Circle if you Moderately Disagree with the statement.
SD - Circle if you Strongly Disagree with the statement.

STATEMENTS	LEVEL OF AGREEMENT				
1. Intimacy and emotional involvement should accompany sexual activity.	SA	A	N	D	SD
2. Sex education should be taught in the public schools.	SA	A	N	D	SD
3. Young people in their reproductive years should have access to contraceptive information and birth control methods.	SA	A	N	D	SD
4. Therapeutic abortions should be available to any woman who desires to terminate a pregnancy.	SA	A	N	D	SD
5. Midwifery and other alternative birthing methods should be available to prospective parents.	SA	A	N	D	SD
6. Childhood sexual experimentation should be viewed as a normal and valuable psychosocial developmental experience.	SA	A	N	D	SD
7. Premarital coitus is acceptable when two people love each other.	SA	A	N	D	SD

		SA	A	N	D	SD
8.	Sexual fantasy should be regarded as a normal and sexually enhancing activity.	SA	A	N	D	SD
9.	Masturbation is an acceptable and healthy form of solitary sexual behavior.	SA	A	N	D	SD
10.	Oral-genital sexual stimulation is neither deviant nor repugnant.	SA	A	N	D	SD
11.	Sexual partners should be willing to try new sexual behaviors.	SA	A	N	D	SD
12.	Extramarital sexual intercourse is permissible under certain situations.	SA	A	N	D	SD
13.	Sexual orientation (preference) should not be a condition for employment, housing, or service (military, ministry).	SA	A	N	D	SD
14.	Prostitution should be decriminalized.	SA	A	N	D	SD
15.	There should be a law to protect women from marital rape.	SA	A	N	D	SD
16.	The penalties for rape should be more equitably applied.	SA	A	N	D	SD
17.	Sexual harassment at work should be against the law.	SA	A	N	D	SD
18.	Pornography should be more clearly defined.	SA	A	N	D	SD
19.	Religion should not get involved with the morality of sexual behavior between adults.	SA	A	N	D	SD
20.	Any activity engaged in by consenting adults, that harms no one, and that is done out of the sight of unwilling viewers, should not be regulated by law.	SA	A	N	D	SD

Answers to Pretest and Posttest Knowledge Questions (Part One)

Pretest Answers

1.	T	21.	b
2.	F	22.	b
3.	T	23.	a
4.	F	24.	d
5.	T	25.	a
6.	T	26.	c
7.	F	27.	d
8.	F	28.	d
9.	T	29.	c
10.	F	30.	b
11.	F	31.	c
12.	T	32.	a
13.	F	33.	c
14.	F	34.	a
15.	F	35.	c
16.	T	36.	b
17.	T	37.	b
18.	T	38.	a
19.	T	39.	c
20.	T	40.	d

Posttest Answers

1.	T	21.	a
2.	T	22.	a
3.	T	23.	b
4.	T	24.	b
5.	F	25.	c
6.	T	26.	c
7.	F	27.	c
8.	F	28.	b
9.	F	29.	d
10.	F	30.	d
11.	F	31.	a
12.	T	32.	a
13.	T	33.	d
14.	F	34.	a
15.	T	35.	d
16.	F	36.	d
17.	F	37.	b
18.	T	38.	a
19.	T	39.	a
20.	T	40.	c

Scoring Knowledge Change:

A. Total Knowledge Score on Posttest ______

B. Total Knowledge Score on Pretest* ______

Knowledge Change ______ (subtract B from A)

*If Pretest score is higher than the Posstest score, the change would be in a negative direction. (We hope that won't be the case!)

Scoring Attitude Change:

Place an "X" for choice on each statement on Pretest and an "0" for choice on Posttest.

Example:

Statement Number	SA	A	N	D	SD
1		0		X	
2	0		X		

Statement Number	Topic	SA	A	N	D	SD
1	bio-psychosocial					
2	cultural-historic					
3	contraception					
4	abortion					
5	childbirth					
6	developmental					
7	love					
8	fantasy					
9	solitary sex					
10	heterosexual					
11	heterosexual					
12	extramarital					
13	homosexuality					
14	sexual variance					
15	sexual assault					
16	sexual assault					
17	sexual harassment					
18	sexual themes					
19	religion					
20	legal					

Was there a change on any specific topic? Yes _____ No _____.

If Yes, which one(s)? To what do you attribute the change?

Was there any overall trend in the direction of attitude change?

How do you feel about the changes that have occurred?